Tooth Decay

Heal Your Teeth and Prevent Cavity Naturally

(The Most Effective Way to Cure and Prevent Cavities at Home)

Susan Grayson

Published By **Darby Connor**

Susan Grayson

Tooth Decay: Heal Your Teeth and Prevent Cavity Naturally (The Most Effective Way to Cure and Prevent Cavities at Home)

ISBN 978-1-77485-451-8

Legal & Disclaimer

The information contained in this book is not designed to replace or take the place of any form of medicine or professional medical advice. The information in this book has been provided for educational and entertainment purposes only.

The information contained in this book has been compiled from sources deemed reliable, and it is accurate to the best of the Author's knowledge; however, the Author cannot guarantee its accuracy and validity and cannot be held liable for any errors or omissions. Changes are periodically made to this book. You must consult your doctor or get professional medical advice before using any of the suggested remedies, techniques, or information in this book.

Upon using the information contained in this book, you agree to hold harmless the Author from and against any damages, costs, and expenses, including any legal fees potentially resulting from the application of any of the information provided by this guide. This disclaimer applies to any damages or injury caused by the use and application, whether directly or indirectly, of any advice or information presented, whether for breach of contract, tort, negligence, personal injury, criminal intent, or under any other cause of action.

You agree to accept all risks of using the information presented inside this book. You need to consult a professional medical practitioner in order to ensure you are both able and healthy enough to participate in this program.

TABLE OF CONTENTS

Introduction

Dear Reader,

This book provides practical steps and strategies on how to stop teeth decay, and to maintain good dental hygiene. I consider that teeth are among the most vital components of our body. Teeth are not only the first thing we see whenever we meet someone, but they also serve as an indicator of how well we treat our own health. There are times when there are external causes outside the control of us that can cause our teeth to become unhealthy. Poor flossing, genetics, brushing habits, or intake of cigarettes and sodas can be a couple of of the factors that can affect the condition of our teeth. The result? The result? Yellow-tinted, stained teeth that over time could result in plaque accumulation and then pain-inducing tooth decay. That can result in increased dental costs and discomfort in the dentist's chair. Everyone hates the idea of having to pay more for dental services.

This is among the reasons mentioned above that I decided that it was the right the right time to study the most effective, efficient and safe methods to avoid tooth decay throughout your life. This book is a reliable guide for avoiding the discomfort and high costs for having whiter, more sparkling teeth for the rest of your life. It is my wish that this book will provide you with all the details you require on how to keep your dental health as well as how to achieve a healthier overall smile. Thank you for geting this book, and I hope you'll thoroughly enjoy it!

Chapter 1: Anatomy Of The Teeth

It is widely known that teeth play an vital function within the mouth. In addition to eating food, they enable us to speak certain words and speak completely. In the west one of the signs of youthfulness is healthy, sparkling teeth. If teeth are damaged within the mouth of a person it is common that this can impact eating and speech negatively.

Teeth are essential to maintaining a healthy mouth's health and, therefore, require regular cleansing. The dental anatomy is usually affected when there are decay process occurring in the teeth. It is important to note as the primary reason behind the brown coloring of teeth. It can also cause cracking and breaking of teeth.

The structure of one tooth contains four main parts: enamel dentin, pulp, the cementum. The dentin and the enamel form the crown of teeth. The other side the root of teeth is made up of pulp and the cementum. They join and secure teeth to jaws. It is essential to be aware of this in order to understand how our teeth function and that something isn't the way it should be.

The enamel is the exterior covering of teeth. It's composed of the mineralized exterior part of the teeth. It is made up of calcium and the phosphorus.

Dentin is the part that is mineralized of teeth. It's the second layer following the enamel. The pulp is the portion of teeth below the dentin and is home to numerous the blood vessels as well as nerves. The teeth's roots are mineralized, and are covered with a substance called cementum. The teeth are anchored by their roots to the jaw bone structure which includes both the upper and lower jaws of the mouth.

The enamel may also suffer from imperfections as a result of the malnutrition that is not adequate. This could lead to demineralization of the teeth and allow decay to develop within the teeth.

It is now known that tooth decay could be an opportunistic dental infection. The infection will benefit from the lack of hygiene in the mouth and teeth which can lead to tooth decay.

If you are suffering from dental problems teeth must be removed and , sometimes, filled in the event of cracks. This exposes the cavities of teeth to further serious infections that if not treated could lead to impairing of your jaws. The infection spreads into the blood stream via the blood vessels of the teeth, in turn, causes damage to the nerves of the jaws and teeth. The nerve damage can be seen in the discomfort that one experiences throughout the day until it is addressed or eliminated.

Deontologists have demonstrated that teeth have the capability of healing themselves naturally. This is only possible when the correct diet is provided to the body in order to improve the development and growth of teeth. This is done by eating an enriched diet that is rich with calcium, phosphorus and calcium in order to ensure the health of the teeth. They help in the demineralization of enamel and dentin. They also aid in the introduction of an additional layer of dentin and enamel.

In the next chapter, I would like you to have a complete understanding of your teeth prior to we begin to discuss ways to stop and treat tooth decay. Chapter 2 will discuss how the medical issues in your teeth started and how they affect the society at large currently.

Chapter 2: Dental Conditions And Medical Conditions Teeth

Tooth decay was first identified in conjunction with finding Vitamin D. In the end, it was found that the absence of Vitamin D was the primary reason for rickets in both women and men. It was also discovered that nutrition is a major element in the health of teeth, and the primary structure of teeth. Simply said healthy teeth are immune to decay and cavities. But, there are many other things that could be taken care of to maintain the best oral health over time.

The most crucial step you could take is to clean your teeth every day to remove acids and sugars that accumulate in the tooth's enamel. This can also help reduce the oxidation of teeth.

Another reason the tooth is becoming a larger issue is that the population is exposed to Fluoride in their water sources and in their food. Fluoride is toxic and can cause various adverse consequences.

Therefore, in order to prevent the buildup of fluoride in your body it is advised to use a water purifier and stay clear of foods that have high levels of fluoride. The most high-fluoride food items include grape juice, pickles tomatoes in canned form and carrots.

Tragically, once consumed the fluoride is absorbed by the body through numerous sites like those in GI, Lungs and Skin. Fluorides that are absorbed are stored within the bones and teeth. Fluoride is eliminated through the kidneys sweat glands, sweat glands, as well as the GI tracts.

Treatment for tooth decay

Although consuming fluoride has been proven to be a risk however, cleaning your teeth using products that contain fluoride are an entirely different matter. The application of fluoride to teeth, either via mouthwashes or toothpastes has been suggested to prevent tooth decay in teeth which are about to erupt.

Its mechanism for action of fluorine in the reduction of dental decay and cavities has been proven to block enzymes that facilitate the oxidation process of food items in the mouth. Furthermore, it reduces microbes' activity, reducing the anaerobic respiration , thereby preventing glycolysis in the mouth as well as on the surface of the teeth that are covered that are covered with sticky food residues.

Common Dental Conditions

The dental Caries is a very common dental disease that affects thousands of patients. The chronic condition is caused by active agents that are part of the oral flora that is indigenous.

Caries lesions are caused by the dissolution of dentin and mineral enamel through the production of acids during the digestion of food residues microorganisms that colonize the tooth surface.

The ions of fluoride are among the minerals that have been shown without doubt to have a negative impact on dental caries in both humans as well as lab animals. The mechanisms that work with fluoride aren't fully understood yet.

In the end, it is noted that fluoride can cause osteomalacia through interfering with the bone mineralization in the osteoid. It increases the chance of fractures to the limbs, and is not recommended to treat of osteoporosis.

There is no single method to stop the development of caries and its progress is available today. It is best to practice an optimal oral hygiene routine in order to minimize the microbial causes of caries agents. Here's a list of five important habits to adopt immediately to improve the hygiene of your mouth.

The teeth should be cleaned for at least two minutes every morning and evening. If you're having difficulty brushing this long, you can try to sing your favorite "ABC's" into your mind in a slow manner until you reach "Z".

After you brush, remember to floss. As easy as it is to floss but many of us don't realize that it's the most crucial aspects of maintaining healthy and strong teeth. Personally, if you're having difficulty with flossing, I recommend these new sticks of floss that recently been released. They're easy to use and aren't as difficult in wrapping the floss between your hands.

After flossing, I suggest using a mouthwash that is alcohol-based. When I asked a variety of physicians, all suggested alcohol-based mouthwashes on the assumption that alcohol itself is used to cleanse your mouth from any extra impurities that are left behind.

Eliminating the fluoride from your drinking water is the most effective method of decreasing dental caries. Systemic fluoride is far more effective in reducing lesions that affect the incisors as well as the soft lingual and buccal surfaces. It is also less effective for cavities and fissures by using inert polymers to stop the development of new lesions.

Modifying your eating habits like cutting down on the amount of food eaten between meals, and avoiding foods that contain sugar, it can make a difference. Replace snacks such as those with fruits , vegetables and cheese, or even nuts is a better choice. Additionally, cut down on the amount of tea, coffee or soft drink. If you have to consume these drinks, treat your teeth well and rinse your mouth after drinking these drinks.

Chapter 3: Diets That Cause Dental Decay

This is a list of food items I have compiled which have been proven to make your teeth unhealthy. These ingredients can be found in a variety of foods and must be avoided at all cost. They can cause tooth decay by decaying your teeth from within and can cause a deterioration of your teeth every day. They also contain enzymes, which help to accelerate the decay of food. Additionally, they contain sugars that stick to teeth, causing the teeth to decay and turn rotten in time. But, brushing your teeth frequently can prevent most of the damages. So, without further delay this is a list of food and drink products you should stay clear of in order to have good teeth in the long run.

Sugars

There are many sugar varieties that can cause tooth decay. They include brown, white organic, cane corn, and jams that contain sugar. The mouth is home to naturally occurring bacteria, known as streptococcus. The bacteria love to feast on sugar and, once it has done so break it down into acids , which destroy tooth enamel. This is an unforgiving situation for those who want sparkling and white teeth since over time, the enamel breaks down substantially.

Grain Products

The grain products are made up of starch and other ingredients that stick to teeth if they aren't washed promptly after eating. The grain products could comprise white sifted flour from maize, wheat sifted flour organic flours. A majority of the items that are made using unsoaked grains aren't good for your teeth.

The products made from these grains include white bread, biscuits, crackers cake, doughnuts and cakes pastas, cookies, muffins and tortillas as well as desserts. In the event of a substitute I suggest buying whole wheat breads because they contain more nutritious grains that don't cause as much harm to your teeth. You can, in the end, be able to eat these kinds of foods so long as you clean your teeth frequently and floss regularly.

Hydrogenated Oils

The majority of margarine and fats are hydrogenated foods. Additionally, there are also poor quality vegetable oils such as soybeans canola, sunflower, and soybean. The hydrogenation process of fats isn't good for our teeth as they cause decay and weakening exactly like sugar or junk food.

Junk Food

The majority of "junk food" nowadays contains hydrogenated oils sugar that are the main cause for tooth decay. Potato Chips soft drinks, potato chips and cheeseburgers could all be classed as "junk foods". Avoid them as much as you can because the fats, sugars, and oils cling onto your teeth. They are difficult to clean. However, as I stated earlier, if you have to indulge in junk food, give your teeth a break and clean your teeth after eating these.

Drinks and Substances

Many drinks that stain your teeth like the coffee drink, drinks with flavor and food additives are among the most common teeth decay causes. Soymilk, proteins, as well as tofu must be avoided when your teeth are not in good health.

Additionally, it needs been proven that the use of substances like cigarettes, alcohol and other alcohol and other drugs can cause tooth decay. I'd like to specifically emphasize smoking as a primary cause of dull and yellow teeth. This bad habit may be the most damaging habit that can lead to tooth decay.

Certain medications have been proven to cause tooth decay, as they strip specific elements found in teeth (including the majority of prescription drugs and vaccines).

Chapter 4: The Foods That Heal And Help Protect Teeth From Decay

It is already known that teeth are able to repair themselves. They only happen in the context of a healthy nutrition and a diet that promotes the development and growth of the teeth inside the mouth.

The function of nutrients is to stimulate the remineralization process of enamel as well as facilitating the creation of dentin. Dentin is created due to the work of the specialized cells that reside in the teeth, known as the odontoblasts.

Nutrition and its effects of nutrition on dental health have been studied for a long time. It is also known that teeth also heal after being damaged by dental caries or attrition. The process is triggered as a particular response to injuries to teeth. The reaction is coordinated by dental odontoblasts within the pulp of teeth. This encourages the development of secondary dentine.

Studies on the effects of nutrition for desineralization of the body under various conditions have been carried out. The results have revealed that the development of secondary dentine is initiated in terms of quality and quantity through the supply of nutrients required to form dentine by odontoblast cells. It has been proven to function independently and is not connected to the tooth's original structure. Studies of dogs fed abundant sources such as these have demonstrated that dentine is extensively laid down.

However, a the diet that was primarily based on grains and vitamins D were poor in calcification, yet, despite the formation of a very little primary dentine. It has been suggested these are the same elements which promote the development of human teeth too.

The factors that encourage the development of teeth are:

The minerals calcium and phosphorus make up the primary minerals found in our diets that help to maintain and improve the health of teeth.

Furthermore fat-soluble vitamin D can an essential element in the development of tooth-forming ordontoblasts.

Mineral absorption inhibitors can include minerals like phytic acids

Similar studies have been conducted on children with dental decay. The study was conducted on children with tooth decay.

The children were grouped into different groups in the study.

A group of people who were fed normal diet had oatmeal that contained an extremely high amount of Phytic Acid in the meal.

The group was fed a normal diet and supplemented with vitamin D.

They were fed an all-gluten diet in addition, added vitamin D.

For the group in which I was there was evidence that the presence of cereal oatmeal increased the amount of dental cavities. Oats are believed to have diminished the ability to absorb of mineral ions.

For the other group the addition of vitamin D helped to improve the healing of cavities. Very few additional cavities developed during the course of treatment.

The third group showed the most notable effect by helping to heal nearly all cavities within the teeth. In addition only a few cavities developed in the mouth.

It was discovered that grains are the most likely contributors in tooth decay. There is a high concentration of Phytic Acid was also suggested as a factor in taking in all mineral ions. It is also believed that another mechanism might be responsible for the development of tooth decay.

The reduction in carbs helps decrease the amount of tooth cavities that are present in the mouth. Additionally, the inclusion of green vegetables and milk in the diet can help aid in the healing of cavities during growth three.

Certain areas of caries of the the teeth were hardened in the diet with higher levels than the minerals salts, such as calcium, phosphorus and calcium. The high content of minerals that calcified stopped the decay and accelerated the healing process.

The process of healing involves creation of a strong layer of enamel that is known as the second denture.

The findings of this study suggest the importance of a diet that contains significant amounts of calcifying components. This includes calcium ions the phosphorus, and vitamin D. This is the amazing secret behind the formation of teeth that are found in the mouth.

He evaluated the effectiveness of the same diet, with the same ingredients, in the curing process of tooth decay.

They were tested with children in the early years and provided with nutritious meals daily and their growth was tracked. The nutritious mix included the consumption of tomatoes and orange juice, as well as a mix of natural vitamins utilizing cod liver, in addition as a pinch of green vegetables was also employed in the production process. Meat stew was used specifically derived from bone marrow, the minced meat that was finely chopped. Yellow carrots were incorporated into the diet to supply an array of the lipid-soluble vitamin A. 2 glasses of milk were also served in the course of the study to children. The diet was changed periodically in order to accommodate the various nutritional requirements, while providing the same food items through the duration of the study.

The approach used for evaluating of the changes that occurred in the evolution of the teeth's formula was documented by x-ray photography to show the modifications in the calcification of the teeth

The presence of mineral phytic acid within the food can act it from being a source of mineral ions and thus decreasing the bioavailability for the mineral that is required for dental calcification process through the diet.

The milk content in the diet that is specially designed to aid in the calcification of teeth can increase the level in calcium ions.

Another significant finding is that there is a high level of Vitamin K2 is an essential vitamin needed for the development of teeth and bone. It is now established scientifically that Vitamin D with Vitamin K2 assists in improving dental and skeletal health for both animals and humans too.

Therefore, a mixture of both diets could be used to make a healthy diet that helps in the healing of teeth and bones within the body.

The components that have been found to help strengthen teeth and improve enamel formationinclude:

Animal products like meat, fish, milk eggs, and other fish..

Utilization of fermented grains, like cereal crackers, oats,

There is a small amount of beans, that contain significant amounts of phytic acid which act as mineral ions sinks. In the event that beans must be used, they'll require overnight soak prior to use for their nutritional value.

The source of starch should be sweet potatoes.

Consume one fruit a day. Sweets that are refined and drinks are to be abstained from.

Vegetables that are used must be steam-cooked and then steamed.

Do not consume industry-related processed food items.

This combination of diet could boost the amount of mineral ions in addition, fat-soluble vitamin D.

This is the most effective combination of diet and lifestyle to help lower the amount of mouth cavities whether it's just at least once or twice per day in your diet.

It is recommended that individuals are capable of brushing their teeth every day.

The teeth should be cleaned and flossed daily after a period of. This will help lower the risk of dental disease.

This method is ideal for those who steal at a early age as they are can only have small amounts of cavities.

It is recommended to consult your dentist specialist before implementing this diet.

Chapter 5: Experienced Tips For Whiter And More Radiant Smile

There are a myriad of tips to manage dental caries and decay. Through my studies I discovered a lot of contradictions between what works and what's urban myth. In the present world, what was once simple is constantly being challenged, making our current systems more effective. So, without further delay I will share the top nine suggestions I discovered in regards in preventing decay of teeth and keep your teeth healthy.

1. Sugar can increase the formation of cavities.

However, this is not the case; sugars don't contribute to the development teeth decay. However, the acids present within the mouth are responsible for most of the process that causes the process of tooth decay. It's also been proven that sugars as well as other carbohydrates increases the chance of developing dental decay or cavities.

2. Acid promote tooth decay

It is well-known there is a fact that acids in the mouth can cause tooth decay. It damages the enamel of teeth, which exposes dentine that can be also eroded, ultimately, opening the pulp. They facilitate the passage of microbes inside the teeth to blood vessels, also cut off the tooth's innervation.

It has been proven that the bacteria that live in the mouth that process sugars are the ones responsible for the production of acids that breakdown teeth formula.

Consuming beverages that contain sugar should be avoided because they encourage the process of tooth decay when they are consumed frequently.

3. Children are more likely to developing cavities.

The majority of toothpastes contain fluorine, which is essential in reducing the incidence for tooth decay specifically for children. Furthermore, the dental cavities that children develop can be repaired when the milk teeth are lost and develop permanent teeth.

4. Aspirin is not the ideal option for toothache.

It is not advised to apply Aspirin when it is placed near the tooth. The most effective method to use Aspirin is to swallow it in order for it to be into the bloodstream to exert its effects at the appropriate points of the body. Aspirin is very acidic , and can increase the effect of tooth decay when it is used in the body.

5. The replacement of fillings is highly recommended.

The fillings in dental teeth will be temporary, and could be only able to last for a short time. They can, however, last for over a longer time as long as your dental hygiene is properly maintained. So, it is suggested that the fillings be replaced when healing has taken place since they could be breeding grounds for bacteria.

6. It is not difficult to determine whether you've created cavities.

The formation of the dental cavity can be an ongoing process that may never be identified until the tooth is already impacted within the pulp. The signs of this could be severe tooth pain. Consult your dentist to help with this. It is therefore suggested to conduct regular dental exams to ensure that you are able to assess the condition of the teeth.

7. Treatment is the best choice to treat tooth decay that is serious

Treatment of the tooth decay would be the most effective alternative since it cuts off the decay process right in the buds. Proper care of your teeth following treatment will aid in managing the process. Be sure to consult your dentist with lots of questions on how to maintain your teeth following treatment. This is to ensure that this will be the final time treating your teeth to treat tooth decay.

8. Most cavities form between the teeth.

The bacteria discover places that could allow them to shield themselves from the effects of brushing and flossing. In many instances they get between teeth, in a way that makes it difficult to remove them when brushing.

A mouthwash that contains alcohol is a great option to ensure that the mouthwash is washed in areas that the toothbrush might not have access to. Consult your dentist about the best type of mouthwash.

9. Clenching and grinding may lead to Cavities

The teeth grinding process may not cause dental cavities; similarly, clenching does not have impact on the teeth. This could lead to cracks or fractures in the teeth, however cavities require a long-lasting process. The enamel is very tough and needs an acidizing substance in order to reduce it. Only bacteria that produce acid can cause this to teeth. Cracks and fractures could encourage rapid growth of tooth decay and cavities.

Chapter 6: Easy Solutions To Prevent Dental Decay

Knowing how to take better care of teeth and gums is essential to ensure the dental health of your teeth are well-maintained. You must learn to stay away from sugary foods like sodas and sweets. Tooth need regular flossing, brushing, and mouthwash in order to stay healthy over the long term. If you concentrate on doing these three thingsevery day you'll see the condition of your teeth dramatically improve. Do not think of this as an obligation, or as something that's uncomfortable, consider the healing process occurring to your teeth and the money you'll be saving by avoiding costly dental appointments. The most important factor that contributes to the dental decay lies in the way of life which one decides to lead.

Cheese Aids Teeth

It has been proven in research that casesin could be beneficial in the protection and preventing tooth decay. It is just so is that among the most potent sources of casein is cheese. While some advise to stay clear of gluten and dairy at all cost I'm here to tell you that casein is beneficial to prevent tooth decay.

Studies have also demonstrated that cheese consumption can increase the amount of calcium present in the mouth. In fact, the presence of calcium saliva plays a significant role in the remineralization of teeth and reducing the likelihood of developing tooth decay.

Sugar-free Chewing Gum

The sugar-free chewing gum is recommended to people suffering from tooth decay or dental cavities. It is because it is made up of an ingredient that is referred by the name of Xylitol. This particular ingredient in sugar-free gum was developed to stop tooth decay. This is due to the fact that Xylitol does not aid in the metabolism of bacteria. Bacteria are unable to metabolize the sugar in order to grow, and thus reduce salivary acidity.

Acid can trigger the development of cavities. The usage of Xylitol is extremely efficient in the production mint. Therefore, next time you go to the supermarket or at the gas station, look for the sugar-free chewing gum that has Xylitol in order to keep your teeth healthy.

Sugar-free Candy

The use of sugar-free candy is a proven method of not harm the teeth , as it can encourage the formation of dental cavities. They are a significant source of dental cavity prevention capabilities. The majority of candy's also contain the unique sugar "xylitol" and include several Lollipops as well as many hard candies. They can assist in the prevention of tooth decay and cavities.

Don't drink Red Wine

The red wine is believed to have teeth staining properties. But, the chemical component found in both white and red wines helps fight bacteria which cause dental decay and cavities.

Eat Raisins

Raisons are believed to behave in the same manner as white and red wine. They contain chemical compounds are flavonoids and polyphenols, which can fight oral bacteria that can cause the development of cavities. There isn't much information to confirm this conclusion and it is highly recommended to consult your physician prior to using this compound to prevent the development of tooth decay and cavities.

Use Straws

Using a straw for drinking a soda or other type of drink that is sugary assists in reducing the point of contact between sugars with your teeth. This is the conclusion of research that was conducted at the University of Philadelphia. It's also more hygienic to drink from a straw instead of drinking directly from bottles of soda.

Dental Sealants

Dental sealants are used to create a protective layer to the surface of back teeth. This is a recommendation from numerous dentists as a good method of preventing tooth decay and the formation teeth cavities. Particularly, the bite teeth's surface is one of the ones that are most susceptible to decay. If there are fractures, cracks or fissures. Many bacteria can be able to hind and serve as a source of bacteria. This is especially true with regards to the crevices in the tooth. Sealants for teeth therefore offer better cover to prevent tooth decay. They also prevent the tooth from getting into and growth in cracks and speeds up the tooth decay process.

Chapter 7: Are You Ready To Treat Tooth Decay & Gum Disease?

When people think of the possibility of tooth decay they tend to blame the problem to poor dental hygiene. But the reality is that gum disease are a result of more than just an ineffective practice of oral hygiene. If you're trying to build good gums and teeth There are several crucial steps to do to reverse the effects of tooth decay.

This book will go over the steps necessary to result in the curing of tooth decay once and all. It also serves as a guideline to help you plan the successful reverse. There are some essential things to consider prior to trying in reversing tooth decay.

Here are some questions to consider asking yourself:

Do you want to prevent tooth decay from happening?

Do you wish to have healthy gums?

Do you want to prevent cavities and other oral health issues?

If you replied positively by saying "yes" in these specific questions, chances are treating tooth decay naturally is the right choice for you. And congrats for making the choice to start working towards achieving your goals by reading this book!

Before we start discussing the steps that are typically required to do to reverse or avoiding tooth decay we will concentrate on a few actions one must consider prior to embarking on this thrilling adventure. Repairing tooth decay is truly the journey that involves the body, the spirit and mind. It's common sense to ensure that you plan your journey before committing to begin.

Here are some tips to help you get going:

1. Brush your teeth.

Cleaning your teeth is a aspect that anyone trying to prevent tooth decay must do. If you're used with brushing your teeth when the time comes to treat tooth decay, it will be something you have already done which is exactly what you require.

2. Floss your teeth after every meal

A crucial aspect of the practice required to prepare you for the curing of tooth decay is to floss your teeth at the end of every meal. If it is a habit to floss following every meal, it helps you to remain in a positive mindset to make the necessary steps that must be taken in order to attain the ultimate goal of reverse tooth decay.

3. Use an occasional tongue scraper every day

One of the most serious errors people commit when planning to heal tooth decay is ignoring in this crucial aspect. If you do not use the tongue scraper at least once per day, it is challenging to reach your objectives. This is because your success is on establishing an effective oral hygiene routine.

As you might imagine, treating tooth decay is more than one day rising to say, "hey, I have an idea that's great I'd like to treat the decay in my teeth and also reverse tooth cavities." Perhaps that is an excellent first step however, to achieve any degree of success in regards to reversing gum disease and tooth decay You must be prepared and be able to achieve success through the steps.

Treating tooth decay A Review

You should realize that you're not the only one around the globe who has aspirations of repairing their tooth decay without aid of dentist. In reality there are millions around the world who would like to reverse teeth decay, and also treat gum disease in a natural way. However, the reality is that only a few people will make the leap and make the decision.

You've been asking yourself "Do you want to prevent dental decay and gum disease from happening at all?" There's a reason why you have to consider this question. People who do not answer this question aren't able to even begin taking any steps to make the process of preventing and reverse tooth decay an actual possibility.

You've already had the opportunity to ask "Do you wish to have healthier gums?" You wouldn't have made it to the next paragraph of this book had you answered no to the question. The truth is that it takes a certain kind to be motivated to accomplish something and a different person to actually accomplish it.

It's awesome to be the kind of person who will take the bull by its horns instead of simply pondering the issue. In general, it can be said that those who tried to treat themselves of tooth decay but had a disastrous failure probably did not fully get their bodies, soul and mind. If you go through all the first questions to determine whether you've got the skills is required to treat your teeth decay on your own you have already a sense of the things you'll need for you to progress.

The process of removing tooth decay is an extremely physical component to it. But any endeavor which you are able to plan ahead for will yield more positive outcomes. It's the same with your mind and the power behind it will lead you to the desired result.

If you look at the people who have reversed their tooth decay in the last few years, or even further back in history that you would like to go, you'll notice a certain thing common for those who have experienced the success they have achieved. They were aware of the process that was involved in the process before diving in and they knew what kind of person they would need to be successful. If you are aware of the kind of person is required to truly commit to curing dental decay and you are aware you are the type of person you are There is anything that can hinder your path and your successful success!

Curing Teeth Decay Step by Step

Once we know what mental state we have to be in to prevent tooth decay, it is time to look over the three essential elements of reverse gum disease and tooth decay naturally.

The first step is to ensure that you're adhering to a healthy lifestyle. This is essential to ensure that you'll succeed in your endeavor to reverse tooth decay. It is logical to consider making a commitment to a healthy lifestyle as this: no one can truly reverse tooth decay unless they commit to a healthier and nutrient-rich diet. It's impossible, this is the reason why this aspect of the procedure is.

Don't believe that you can continue eating the wrong diet if wish to reverse tooth decay or gum diseases. To reverse tooth decay, you need to be determined and motivated and that means you have to be determined to eat nutritious food that is high with fat-soluble nutrients and mineral. You'll notice that the standard diet of America nowadays is high in sugar, grains and starch grains as well as vegetable oils. It is also lacking in healthy fats and fat-soluble vitamins. This is not what is recommended to ensure good bones and for the prevention of gum and tooth decay disease.

A healthy diet is beneficial for many reasons. It is one of the reasons it consistently leads to feeling more confident about your self. If you're missing this essential piece of advice then it's difficult to reverse tooth decay. In addition, following an enlightened diet can result in a better the health of your bones and preventing further tooth decay, while also enhancing the body's ability to heal dental cavities and other issues.

Additionally, implementing a proper dental hygiene routine is vital in order to reverse tooth decay. There are numerous advantages to this, but when we examine the pertinent benefits in terms of treating tooth decay, stopping further tooth decay will be considered to be essential. If you don't prevent further dental decay and cavities it is next to difficult to reverse the effects of tooth decay.

Other benefits of implementing an effective oral hygiene regimen in relation to preventing tooth decay are the prevention of gingivitis as well as stopping the accumulation of plaque. If you're not taking steps to stop the accumulation in plaque could be difficult to achieve everything related to the prevention of gum disease and cavities.

After spending the time and effort to commit you to an energizing lifestyle and following a proper dental hygiene routine You may think that you're in a position to get rid of the decay in your teeth. Even if you're not sure make sure you know if you are really prepared or if your thoughts are pushing you into believing that you're at ease. Most those who achieve natural tooth decay reverse find that they need to prepare themselves for a complete change in their attitude, diet and way of life. .

In the final phase of the process of preparation ensure that you focus your efforts on taking vitamin as well as mineral supplementation. It's easy to ignore this element of good oral health. However, when you focus your efforts on this specific element you'll discover that you can improve your dental health and reverse dental cavities. Additionally taking minerals and vitamins can help you to avoid mineral deficiencies within your body and prevent osteoporosis.

In no time you've committed yourself to a balanced diet and following a proper routine for oral hygiene and taking vitamin or mineral-rich supplements you'll be in a position to stop tooth decay without the assistance from a professional. In most cases, it requires a time of preparation and commitment to be fully prepared but this time of time will pass soon enough. If you are able to find the determination to reverse tooth decay, begin by committing yourself to a balanced diet and setting up a proper dental hygiene regimen. You'll find that your body, mind and mind are fully prepared to utilize its natural healing powers to treat gum disease and tooth decay!

Dietary Guidelines to Improve the Health of your mouth and reverse Cavities

Cut out food items that contain Phytic acid. These include beans, grains and nuts. Prior to the time that humans began the cultivation of rice, grains and corn, fossils of human remains suggest dental decay wasn't an everyday occurrence.

Reduce the amount of food which contain starches or sugars (even naturally occurring sugars). You should not only eliminate starch and sugar but also cut down on your starchy and fruit consumption. A good example of a starchy vegetable are sweet potatoes. Instead, you should eat the minerals rich foods like meats, vegetables as well as healthy fats. Bone broths have a significant quantity of minerals and make a great supplement to the healthy food plan.

Eat a lot in healthy fats. It is important to consume an eating plan that is rich in nutritious meats like fish, organic beef chicken, venison and so on. Ideally, it is recommended to include a cup of unprocessed organic coconut oil into your diet. You can substitute vegetable oil with this wonderful healthy oil that is healthy for every meal.

In essence, the diet that aids in tooth decay prevention is devoid of grains and beans, as well as nuts and without processed sugar and has a tiny amount of starches and fruits. Additionally, it is recommended to be eating plenty of minerals-rich vegetables proteins, healthy fats, as well as mineral-rich bone broth.

Vitamins and Supplements to improve oral health and reverse Cavities

In order to aid your body's regeneration process of cavities and bones and cavities, you can boost the mineral content of your body by taking supplementation with vitamins and other supplements. Although a balanced diet that is low in Phytic acid might be sufficient however, the majority of natural food items sold in the stores today are deficient of essential nutrients because of the deficient soil they're grown in. So, supplementation with other supplements could aid in resolving the deficiency of nutrients in food. To accelerate your process of getting remineralized you'll need to consume Fermented Cod Liver Oil as well as High Vitamin Butter Oil daily. I will explain the reasons:

Fermented Cod Liver Oil

The fermented cod liver oil rich in healthy fats as well as Omega-3. It is crucial to reverse and stopping tooth decay. The oil is available in capsule form or liquid form. As the absence in fat-soluble vitamins are the primary reason behind tooth decay, it is essential to make sure that you're receiving sufficient amounts of Vitamin A in addition to Vitamin D. Cod liver oil fermented is high in both, and can be consumed daily to prevent tooth decay and tooth decay. Fun fact 1 teaspoon of cod liver fermented oil contains as much Vitamin D equivalent to 21 grams of whole milk, (or 60 eggs!).

Butter Oil

Butter oil is a rich source of an hormone that is similar that of Vitamin D that is found in the milk of animals fed on grass. When combined with cod's fermented liver oil on a daily basis it acts in conjunction with Vitamin A as well as Vitamin D to quickly help the body begin the process of remineralization.

You can now take the two supplements on their own or you can buy the two supplements Fermented Cod Liver Oil and

Butter Oil in one bottle! We suggest Blue Ice Royal Butter Oilor Fermented Cod Liver Oil Blend. Read some reviews and then make the choice which is the best fit for your needs.

Additional Supplements

Coconut Oil

Pure, unrefined and organic coconut oil is a great source of beneficial fats as well as fat-soluble vitamins that have been discussed before are essential to maintaining healthy oral health. You can not only include this in your diet to improve your oral health, but you also can engage in oil pulling, which involves swirling coconut oil around the mouth for about 15 minutes to eliminate contaminants from the body. Oil pulling is a wonderful supplement to a healthy diet and has many benefits to your body! For more information about oil pulling, read the Coconut Oil Detox Diet

Chapter 8: Guidelines To Be Considering When Trying To Prevent And Reverse Tooth Decay

The process of reversing tooth decay requires being well-informed, healthy and motivated. A lot of times, these characteristics are able to be uncovered from those who follow specific rules observed that help to draw out the particular traits. This section will explore some of the guidelines that were developed specifically to aid in successful cavity and gum disease reverse.

If you're committed to a healthy lifestyle and lifestyle, it is essential to incorporate the correct amounts of nutrients in the diet. This will assist the middle of the tooth to regenerate dentin, which is the tooth's layer underneath the enamel. The enamel is then able to regenerate the tooth on the exterior, reverse tooth decay and cavities. This is only one of many positive effects this method will bring about when you are preparing.

Furthermore, you'll be more confident about yourself and increase your bone health, all and prevent any further tooth decay. This is especially important when it comes time to stop tooth decay.

In your time of preparation, be aware that people who regularly practice an effective oral hygiene regimen are likely to maintain their flossing routine since it is the most crucial aspect of the dental hygiene regimen. It's amazing how simple steps can be so crucial in the bigger picture. If you consider yourself as healthy and are able to identify the signs of health, it is quite easy to incorporate these guidelines into your routine procedure. Additionally, if you are able to keep up with flossing because it is the most essential part of your oral hygiene routine, it can help to eliminate any food leftovers which contain starches and sugars that are the major causes of dental decay and cavities.

Additionally, we should keep in mind the purpose of taking vitamins or mineral supplements. Most likely, this will require an increased degree of concentration to fully benefit from minerals and vitamins during the process of treating tooth decay. As you work towards the reverse of decay in teeth, elimination of mineral deficiencies and osteoporosis prevention it is important to reduce your intake that you consume of Phytic acid that you are eating, as it is the primary factor in how the body absorbs these vital minerals and vitamins. If you keep this mentality in mind and attitude, you'll allow your body to begin the process of remineralization.

The body absorbs phytic acid through the intake of cereals, seeds and nuts as well as legumes and this means you are more prone to having greater rates of teeth decay, deficiency of minerals, and bone problems. If your diet is high with phytic acid you'll discover that you are likely to lack the correct quantity of calcium , phosphorus and calcium that is associated to healthy bone growth.

As you can imagine, it requires a person who is motivated to reach the ultimate objective of reversing tooth decay. Although it's not difficult to prepare and reverse tooth decay it is a testament of it that one need to be committed. Be aware that we're not willing to abandon the cause. Curing tooth decay is not just is about a mental state one is in good health, it is it also means being committed to the task of removing tooth decay.

If you commit to being fully prepared and complete the task, you will see it through! Do you remember when you were asked these questions?

Do you wish to stop tooth decay from happening?

Do you need healthy gums?

Do you want to prevent cavities and other oral health issues?

In all of these scenarios the answer was "yes". This is the reason we've concluded that you're fit committed, enthusiastic and focused on getting rid of your gum disease. These are the traits that will help you achieve success once you have finally cured your tooth decay on your own. Be sure to stick to a healthy lifestyle and follow a regular oral hygiene routine , and also take minerals and vitamins. You'll be on your path to optimal oral health in a flash!

The Curing Tooth Decay Free

People often think it's expensive to spend dollars to treat tooth decay, because you have visit the dentist, buy expensive dental hygiene products, and so on. In reality, it's not that expensive. You can reverse tooth decay at the convenience of your home. If you're trying ways to stop tooth decay no cost, the primary goal you should do is remove any notions of how costly treating tooth decay is likely to cost.

There are three fundamental rules to help you manage your goal of curing tooth decay while also saving money. If you concentrate on options which do not need a large expense, you allow your mind be focused on the most important aspects. Be aware that adhering to a healthy lifestyle and maintaining a proper dental hygiene routine and taking supplements for minerals and vitamins is of the utmost importance. If you adhere to these easy steps, you won't need to see the dentist ever again however, you will be able to treat gum and tooth decay disease, without spending a dime of your hard-earned cash.

There are many options you could take to save amount of money. There is no need to shell out huge sums of money in order to reverse tooth decay. If you think into it, and don't let your feelings dictate choices with any amount of money, you will discover numerous options that are cost-free or inexpensive that are more suitable than more costly alternatives when your goals are your primary goal.

There are many options that are affordable to accomplish the goal to help you manage tooth decay. Before these luxury options were even considered patients were able to treat tooth decay with no balloons and steamers that are commonly associated with more expensive alternatives.

Do you have any idea why indigenous people living without dentists have excellent dental health, no cavities, and do not require braces? It's because they are not able to access processed western foods which we consume in the Western society that is industrialized. Their diets are comprised of raw, natural foods, and meat , which means they consume large quantities of fat-soluble vitamins and minerals and little or no Phytic acid.

The best advice is to make your primary goal the first priority in your head. Making a commitment to a healthy diet, following an effective oral hygiene routine and taking vitamins and mineral supplements are the thing you need to be focusing on. If you look at your actions from a focal point it becomes increasingly easy to identify when you're throwing money away that is not necessary to spend.

Making a commitment to a healthy diet doesn't need a huge amount of money. The aim is to feel more confident about yourself and it is possible to achieve this without breaking the budget. A good oral hygiene routine does not require breaking your budget. It typically requires more money to adhere to a proper routine for oral hygiene. The reason to focus on maintaining a healthy dental hygiene routine is because you will be able to avoid any further decay of your teeth. This is also a good thing, and doesn't require a huge amount of money to accomplish.

Then, you should focus your thoughts on the importance of taking vitamin and mineral supplements and ways to make sure you are taking vitamin and mineral supplements correctly. Do not be enticed by products that demand large sums of money, as there are many options to take vitamins or mineral supplementation that don't require writing large checks.

The bottom line is that if you remain focused on your goals so that you don't spend in excess to reach your goal of preventing tooth decay. There are cheaper alternatives to consider and knowing how your feelings influence your financial decisions can help you manage expenses in the process of preventing tooth decay.

The Cure for Tooth Decay in Everyday Life

Reversing tooth decay is regarded as a way to live. It's something you can incorporate into your life in many ways. When you're working towards preventing tooth decay, it is also possible to examine how this process could influence other areas of your life.

In reality, the solution to stop and reverse tooth decay requires change in how you think. The innate motivation essential for reversing tooth decay can be seen in other aspects in your daily life. In a matter of minutes you'll be displaying your motivation in all you do. This is the good side of naturally repairing tooth decay that many do not see.

It is essential to have the desire to lead a healthier life style to prevent tooth decay and. Another aspect of this can have a profound impact on your life. The more you rely on this quality in yourself to reverse the process of tooth decay naturally and improve your oral health, the more you'll be able to see this quality in other areas of your life.

Curing tooth decay involves more than simply reversing tooth decay. It's an option for your lifestyle in many ways. If you view it as an option for your lifestyle you'll enjoy the benefits of excellent oral health and an increased attitude to your life . As you could imagine, you need certain qualities to be able to achieve the goals up to the final. It's common sense to let all these benefits to be utilized in other aspects of our lives.

Do you remember at the beginning of this book that it was your turn to respond to these questions

Do you wish to stop tooth decay from happening?

Do you need healthy gums?

Do you want to prevent cavities and other oral health issues?

These are choices made in the course of life. These are questions asking you to consider the virtues that determine if you're able to stop tooth decay. If you replied positively by saying "yes" in the previous questions, you weren't only proving you had the physical capacity to heal tooth decay, but instead you were confirming your life.

There is no guarantee that removing tooth decay is an easy job. Each of the rewarding activities requires the form of a devotion. Dental decay treatment isn't an one of them.

If you are committed to the ultimate goals are likely to discover the process of curing tooth decay incredibly satisfying. Congrats on taking the decision to begin this new lifestyle!

Chapter 9: Strategies For Curing

Decay In The Teeth

If you've decided to work towards cure the tooth, there's a variety of methods you can take in order to stop tooth decay in the coming months. Below are a few suggestions that can assist you in the treatment of tooth decay:

The first step in the process of preparing for treating tooth decay included the necessity of adhering to a balanced diet. It is essential that, when you are committed to a healthy lifestyle ensure that you are getting the correct quantity of mineral content in your food. This can help the teeth's center regenerate the dentin layer of tooth that lies beneath the enamel. The enamel is then able to restore its mineralization on the exterior, thus reversing tooth decay and cavities. It is suggested that your diet is free of Phytic acid, and rich in calcium Vitamin D, calcium as well as other vital supplements.

We should be conscious that it is important to follow an effective oral hygiene routine. It is a vital part of preparing for the treatment of tooth decay. It's not easy and the most effective way to overcome this obstacle is to continue flossing since it is the primary element of a regular dental hygiene regimen. It will help remove any leftover food which contain starches and sugars that are the major causes of tooth decay and dental cavities.

It could be a huge difficult task to keep your mind to take vitamin and mineral supplements. However it is crucial to be successful in treating tooth decay that you do this. It can help cut levels that you consume of Phytic acid that you consume, as it affects the way your body is absorbing these essential minerals and vitamins. This will enable your body to begin process of remineralizing your teeth and bones.

If you follow these suggestions to stop tooth decay, you'll realize that you're gaining numerous benefits. Here are some benefits will be noticed once you implement your plan to stop tooth decay.

When you make the commitment to a healthy lifestyle You will feel more confident about your body.

Making a commitment to a healthy diet can also help to improving your bone health and helping prevent tooth decay.

A good dental hygiene routine can help prevent the development of further decay on your teeth.

In addition, a regular routine for oral hygiene can help to prevent gingivitis.

When you begin to take mineral and vitamin supplements you'll find that you're preventing you from developing deficiencies in mineral nutrients which could lead to diseases and chronic illnesses.

Supplementing with vitamins and minerals helps in preventing osteoporosis.

There are many immediate benefits to reverse tooth decay. Improved body's ability to treat dental decay, as well as other issues and preventing the accumulation of plaque are two direct benefits of adhering to a balanced diet and following a proper dental hygiene routine. These benefits will enhance your overall health and well-being beyond just curing tooth decay. Additionally the use of vitamin and mineral supplements aids in improving the condition of your teeth and reverse tooth decay. To reap the full benefit of these benefits, here these guidelines to assist you in reaching your goal of reverse tooth decay.

When you adhere to the guidelines and guidelines in this article then you'll be moving towards the right direction to stop tooth decay. Make sure you allow you time to completely cure the tooth decay. A time frame that is comfortable to prepare yourself for treating tooth decay is crucial to achieve the greatest success.

Chapter 10: Signs Of Tooth Decay

The process of tooth decay is referred to as dental caries is one of the most prevalent dental issues which affects patients all over the globe. While it may appear harmless, can cause tooth loss if not taken care. The most effective way to combat it is to prevent its development, but if it isn't possible to stop it then you must at the very least attempt to spot it in the beginning stages.

The dental procedures developed to fight teeth decay the most efficient when they are carried out at the beginning of the tooth decay. The deeper the penetration , and the more widespread the infection the greater risk is the tooth of having to take urgent actions. To increase your chances to save your teeth you must be aware of the signs of an infection:

* Dark spots or lines on the teeth: Teeth decay is visible clinically on the teeth as spots or lines on the rough and smooth surface of teeth. Healthy teeth are clean and white appearing. Any shadow or

evidence of decayed teeth is a sign of a bacterial infection.

* Pain that originates from the tooth: The pain that results from toothache could or might not be felt following being exposed to stimuli. The most frequent stimuli are sweet or cold foods however, touch and bite can cause discomfort. The degree of discomfort and pain may vary. In certain instances, the symptoms may manifest as constant, dull discomfort, while in other situations, they could be a sensation of stinging that is immediate and intermittent. It could occur like lightning and be debilitating, based upon the extent of issue.

The tooth is a cavity A cavity is a hole or opening inside the tooth. Cavities typically develop in the deep grooves and fissures in teeth, however they can also form over the surface of the teeth. Cavities may be visible or unnoticeable, based on the extent of exposure to the pulp. For shallower depths it is possible to be able to fix a cavity however, when the issue is more serious and the tooth is in a more pronounced state, a root canal or tooth extraction could be the best option.

"Bood odor" There's numerous reasons for your breath to be sour however, dental decay may easily be the cause. Dental decay signifies the presence of decayed or damaged tissues. It could include pus and blood. If there's an oral infection and your breath is smelling bad and smell rotten. This is different from bad breath that comes from the foods you consume because bad breath is eliminated with thorough brushing, washing and flossing. This type of breath odor does not disappear, it's only treated with the proper treatment.

Swollen gums: If tooth decay is serious the infection may be spread to the pulp tissue and the adjacent tissues. This can cause swelling to be visible. Sometimes , the swelling is visible within the gums, however in other instances it can only be seen on a radiograph. The more severe swelling issues may even affect the facial soft tissues and are very noticeable.

• Radiographic luminosity: By using an X-ray or radiograph tooth decay is simpler to detect. In actual there are many not yet diagnosed problems can be detected by a dental radiographs. A radiolucent spot in the tooth can indicate dental cavities.

"Pus" formation is the body's primary defense against infection by bacteria is the release of antibodies. To combat the infection that is present within the mouth area, your body could release antibodies that cause pus to develop. If abscess or pus is present, fever and swelling can be anticipated.

• Unpleasant taste in your mouth Dental decay may cause mouths to have an unpleasant taste. The reason for this could be caused by food that is stuck to teeth, or blood flowing through the soft tissues, pieces of decayed tooth structures and even the presence pus.

If you suspect that any of you are experiencing any of the following symptoms within your mouth and teeth, you should schedule appointments with your dental professional as soon as possible.

What causes tooth decay?

Inside the mouth are dormant bacteria which are harmless when not activated. Plaque forms when the bacteria are allowed to mix with food. This sticky substance releases acid. Although the results that follow do not pose an immediate risk, the constant disregard for your oral health can result in the destruction and possibly loss of the tooth. Dental decay begins at the surface of the tooth - called the enamel. It it spreads to dentin before infecting tissues of the pulp. If the problem is identified earlier it can be dealt with quickly. If the problem is more severe you could be at risk of losing the tooth affected.

As with everything it is helpful to know the cause. If you are aware of the root causes, you will be able to be proactive in preventing tooth decay and improve your chance of avoiding the tooth decay. The first paragraph in this article outlines the vibrant sequence of events that occur within the mouth, which can lead into tooth decay. The causes are explained in greater detail:

1. Insufficient oral hygiene: You're required to take proper dental hygiene practices on a regular basis. In fact everybody is required to clean your teeth at least 3 times per daily, and after each meal. If you fail to follow good oral hygiene habits your risk to develop tooth decay will increase. Cleanse, floss, and brush your mouth with plenty of water to keep the surfaces of your mouth clean and free of plaque.

2. Plaque accumulation occurs within the mouth on an regular basis. Foods that mix with saliva and bacteria creates an impervious white film that covers the teeth. If your attempts to clean your mouth fail to eliminate plaque, it can build up. Plaque that's allowed get a hold of itself will harden and calcify. It causes irritation to tissues, and releases acids that harm the tissues that are hard to the tooth, leading to cavities.

3. Unhealthy diet choices Food choices and drinks can affect the condition that your mouth is in. Foods that contain carbohydrates and sweets as well as drinks must be avoided or diminished since they break into sugars which allow bacteria to flourish and grow within the mouth. The accumulation of sticky foods between and inside the fissures and grooves of the teeth can be a issue. Food can become trapped within these areas which allows bacteria to flourish and get into the teeth.

4. Incorrectly aligned and misaligned teeth. While the placement of teeth can be seen as an aesthetic concern more than anythingelse, incorrectly aligned teeth may also lead to tooth decay due to the fact that the poor arrangement can trap food. Food particles that build up in unwelcome areas can result in caries. The location of teeth can make cleaning them difficult and allow bacteria to take a toll.

5. Dry mouth is a condition that affects the saliva produced in the mouth is supposed to aid in preventing the development of disease by washing food particles out of

the teeth. If the consistency and structure of saliva changes or if there's an insufficient production of saliva the dryness of the mouth can lead to the possibility of developing cavities. These medications and substances may cause dry mouth : tricyclic antidepressants beta-blockers, radiotherapy, anti-psychotics such as antihistamines, anti-epileptics, and antih.

6. Smoking tobacco and cigarettes smoking is generally considered to be a harmful habit. Indirectly affecting the growth of dental decay Smokers are at a greater risk of developing tooth decay because the chemicals present in tobacco and cigarettes reduce saliva production and remove the primary defense to tooth decay.

Simply put, it's bacteria that cause tooth decay. However, since there is an inbuilt population of bacteria living in your mouth it is impossible to label the bacteria as the sole culprit. The level of acidity in a person's saliva may be identified as the cause, however as there is little that could be accomplished to manage the amount of saliva you're consuming so it is more beneficial to concentrate on sugars. Carbohydrate-based food products breakdown into sugars, which create acids that demineralize the tooth structure. If your teeth are properly cleaned tooth decay should not be a problem you need to address.

How to treat it, prevent it, stop it, reverse It...

Dentistry is a vast discipline that includes the detection, prevention treatment, and treatment of various dental ailments. When a patient visits an office for dental care the patient is treated by a highly skilled dental team. All concerns are handled professionally. Any oral problem that is present is evaluated in a way that the most appropriate treatment can be offered. After a series stages, the severity of the dental problem is assessed and the appropriate treatment is suggested.

Prevent of Tooth Decay

The most fundamental solution to teeth decay is to stop the onset of tooth decay. It requires hard effort and determination however, you can endure your whole life without experiencing tooth decay, if you follow these steps:

a. Maintain oral hygiene Time spent in your home can help ensure your dental health. Maintain your mouth's cleanliness by flossing, brushing and rinsing regularly. As it's explained within this guide, the accumulation of plaque could lead to dental infections or dental caries. If you're looking to stop the beginning of illness make sure you are attentive to maintain your mouth's cleanliness. Plaque can cause disease, and if your mouth is free of plaque and healthy, it will remain healthy for a longer period of time.

b. Oral Prophylaxis: Cleaning as well as scaling are the primary fundamental treatment that dentists can offer to stop the accumulation of plaque as well as dental caries. Oral prophylaxis can be prescribed for all patients every six months or once each year. It involves scaling, planning and scraping dental surfaces in order to get rid of any plaque. Based on the amount of plaque, plaque may be detected either supragingivally or subgingivally. Plaque is scraped carefully off the tooth in order to remove it and bring the oral condition back to their normal, healthy.

C. Application of Fluoride: Fluoride helps strengthen the hard tissues of teeth. Teeth that are weaker can be less prone to bacteria by the exposure of fluoride. The fluoride is absorbed through fluoridated water or be applied directly. The application, whether on teeth that are developing or fully grown aids in strengthening the teeth. Teeth that are developing in children are the ideal candidates for protecting against fluoride. Regular doses of fluoride strengthen their teeth, and they won't have to worry about tooth decay throughout their existence.

D. Dental sealants. The sealant can be described as a covering of resin. The material can completely cover the surface of the teeth, including the pits and grooves that are deep. It is like a protective raincoat or a helmet providing protection for the tooth to make it less susceptible to bacterial attack. Dental sealants are applied over the teeth to make the surface more smooth and resistant to infection.

E. Diet Modification It's not an immediate solution to tooth decay, but changing your diet to ensure it's a mix of most dental-friendly ingredients is always a good idea. By abstaining from sweets and eating more nutritious foods and naturally cleans your teeth and nourishing, you will have an uninjured mouth.

The effective prevention of diseases is a joint effort of patients and dentists. The things you do at home as well as the work your dentist puts into to prevent disease will give your mouth a solid first line of defense against infections.

The treatment of tooth Decay

If your efforts for preventing tooth decay do not work and an infection develops, it could and then become a problem. The severity of the condition the appropriate treatment could be one of the following:

a. Dental Filling A filling for a tooth is the most fundamental method of treating decayed teeth. It involves cleaning as well as drilling the teeth in order to remove the affected tissue, and then filling with the right material. The standard direct filling substance is a composite resin that is tooth-colored and amalgam. indirect fillings require laboratory fabrication . They could be made of ceramic porcelain, gold or.

B. Root Canal Treatment: If the tooth infection is more serious and has already spread to tissues surrounding the pulp, then a filling for the tooth is no longer effective. The best way to eliminate the infection is achieved through a pulp treatment. This involves the extrication and removal of pulp in the canals. The root canal proccdure can help to prolong the lifespan of teeth. However, it can make the tooth more brittle, so the restoration with a crown might be necessary.

C. Tooth Extraction: If the tooth no longer able to be saved with the help the use of dental fillings, or an extraction canal, then the tooth can be totally eliminated through extraction. Through the removal of the tooth the infection is eradicated but the tooth gets also removed.

D. Dental Crowns If the destruction of the tooth is more severe and more of the structure is gone because of the tooth infection, a dental cap can be made over the tooth to provide an aesthetic, durable and practical solution. Crowns or caps for dental use are prosthetic alternatives that require a lot of grinding and preparation, however they provide excellent protection for teeth.

If the infection in the mouth is already very severe at the time it is discovered it is always a cause for tooth loss. If a tooth gets removed, it should be replaced, and prosthetics need to be considered in order for the health of the mouth to be repaired. The most common prosthetic choice is removable dentures. Patients may also think about implant-supported dental bridges to make up the gap left by the tooth removed.

Dental Decay is a problem in Babies

From the moment the child's first tooth is removed through their gums they're susceptible to getting tooth decay. Many parents are negligent enough to ignore this fact and are forced to face the pain of their child from a tooth infection in the early years of. The process of dealing with dental cavities by yourself can be difficult, but seeing an insignificant child screaming in pain can be depressing and can be painful to watch.

The vigilance of parents in preventing dental decay within their child's tooth must be of the highest priority. The development of tooth decay is not difficult and, in infants, it is commonly referred to for its dreaded "milk caries." It's named this way due to the fact that milk is the ingredient that is most often involved in tooth decay in infants. Milk is sweet , and it breaks down into sugars that cover the mouth and teeth. Sugars help bacteria thrive and if you're not able maintain your kid's oral healthy, bacteria can grow and take over their teeth.

Cleaning and brushing

The first tooth of a baby appears between 4 and six months, parents are expected to ensure the hygiene of their child's mouth. There are toothbrushes as well as mouthwashes that parents could make use of to keep their baby's mouth healthy. Use the steps below to prevent the formation of milk caries

* Brushing your teeth using either toothpaste or not is important. It is recommended to use toothpaste designed for children as the formula is gentler and more suitable for a child's delicate tissues.

* Do not let your child to go to bed with their bottle of milk. The milk that sits inside the mouth may get stuck to teeth and result in tooth decay. It is recommended to change to a water bottle just before your child goes to sleep in the event that you can't brush their teeth any more. Water can wash away plaque that

has accumulated in the mouth, and also prevent development of caries.

If you're unable to clean or change bottles, it is possible to clean your child's mouth using moist gauze or cotton to eliminate adhering plaque from the lips, lips the tongue, gums and teeth. It is not necessary get your kid up up; you can wash all surfaces to prevent formation of diseases.

The baby and the dentist

From the time an infant is able follow directions and is requested to sit in the chair, they must be brought to see the dentist who is friendly. In some instances, this appointment could involve the child lying down alongside the parent. However, it's only a brief introduce to the dentist. chair, the instruments for dentistry and any other dental procedure that could be carried out.

The bond that develops between children and their dentist from this point on will be extremely beneficial. If you can introduce your toddler to the significance of dental hygiene at an early age, you can make it more of an enjoyable task, and becoming a routine that is able to be kept away from.

Dental decay is a problem occurs in Infants and Children

When the first teeth appear from the mouth The oral cavity of children continues to grow. Through these stages when the responsibility for taking care of teeth is passed by the parent to their child. When the task is completed by the parents, children gradually assumes the responsibility of keeping his teeth clean and free of disease However, only through proper instructions will they succeed.

Dentition Phase: The Mixed Dentition Phase

A person goes through two types of tooth: infant or deciduous ones and the permanent or succeeding ones. As the transition takes place from the baby to permanent teeth, your child is in the mix dentition stage and also given the chance to care for their teeth.

Based on the type of care given to the child while they were young or older, their mouth could be free of disease, however, it could also be afflicted with dental problems and permanent teeth that aren't entirely healthy. First permanent teeth are formed at six years old. If the child is lucky they may already have cavities.

The way that dentist and parents take in these phases will depend on the state that the dental teeth are in.

The Child's Education at the Home

If you wish for your kid to become more accountable with regards to their teeth, then you must dedicate a significant amount hours to education about dental health as well as oral hygiene training. Parents are expected to have an influencer for their children. This should include instruction on oral hygiene and treatment.

There are videos and books you can utilize to help your child learn about gums and teeth. Illustrations can help explain concepts in ways that children can easily be able to comprehend and understand.

* Modeling by example is equally crucial for children. Young people rely on peers

for everything. They admire their parents and mimic what they do, therefore should you wish the child you love to keep careful in their efforts to maintain their oral health You must be an excellent model for them to emulate. "Monkey observe and do" You can be confident that your child will follow the example you set for them.

* If you would like your child to brush their teeth regularly, you could monitor their brushing habits by doing it together. Brush your teeth together with the child, and create a pleasurable brushing session that you are enjoying to make them be looking forward to it for a time they will be able to spend with you.

Introduce the Child to the Dentist

The introduction of your children to the dentist should be taken care of in the early years. Parents make the error of not taking the child in early to the dentist, making the initial visit to the dentist one in which the issue is already addressed.

Ideally, the initial dental visit should be to provide a basic introduction to the dental profession. As the child grows older, the visit may include procedures such as dental cleaning sealing, fluoride application and sealants. However, the rest of the procedures are kept out in order to avoid unpleasant experiences and trauma. It is important to make your child take dental treatment initially, through making them more comfortable with the dentist and dental office. This can be done by following the following:

Bring your child along with you to your dental appointments. A great way to make your child feel more comfortable with the dentist as well as the dental clinic is to take your child with you whenever you schedule an appointment. It is not necessary to explain the procedure to the child. They are able to be in the reception area or observe your visit but what you're doing is showing your child that this isn't something to be scared of and dentists are not a stranger to them.

Discuss with them oral hygiene and dental care. Make it a point to talk about dental hygiene and oral care for your kid. At this stage they're in a position to comprehend things, and you are able to explain the various techniques used in the dental practice to help them understand what they can expect.

* Do not make use of the dentist to make a threat. Parents often employ dentists as a way to get their child to behave. They love making use of dental injections to get their child's attention. Although this can be beneficial, it should be avoided as a large number children are scared of visiting the dentist since they consider dentists frightening and their injections are threatening.

If you take care of things correctly taking your child visiting the dentist first might be an easy task with everything going smoothly. However there are a few parents and their children are fortunate enough to not suffer tooth decay prior to their first visit. If the dental condition is already deteriorating further procedures could be suggested such as teeth extractions and dental fillings and treatment of the pulp. A child might not be as open to these procedures. They can be intimidating as well as demanding and difficult for children to comprehend, which is why going at it normally isn't always feasible.

The most extensive dental procedures for tooth decay can be performed under sedation. The administration of sedation orally, intravenously and via inhalation aids in change the child's perception so that they are able to be relaxed throughout the procedure.

Chapter 11: Tooth Decay For Teens

At this point the teenager's tooth will be in the mixed dentition phase , and their mouth will be comprised of the permanent teeth. Dental hygiene could or might have the oversight of parents, but the practices will be carried out by the person who is doing it. In this stage parents need to trust the base they have laid for the child to look into consideration. If the dental education and model is solid the child will be ready to assume the responsibility of maintaining their dental hygiene However, if the hygiene is poor, they could suffer from dental issues.

A very important habits that a teenager should establish at this point is visiting the dentist regularly. Oral Prophylaxis and dental checks are suggested twice per year or once every six months, to ensure that the beginning of the disease could be avoided and detected earlier.

Teenagers and Orthodontics

Although orthodontic treatment isn't only for teens, most of patients using orthodontic braces are teenagers because dentists are more likely to perform the procedure when they are young. As teens get older there are all the permanent teeth are in place which means that orthodontic treatment can continue. Furthermore the bones are in a growth phase which means that speed and convenience of treatment is possible.

Braces for dental use are fixed to the face of your teeth using an adhesive. Consider that if you change from a totally free mouth you'll have brackets, wires , and rubbers everywhere on your mouth and teeth and mouth, which means hygiene could be an issue.

* If a person is urged to maintain the best oral hygiene practices without braces in order to prevent tooth decay They are likely to be more thorough when braces are in place because food items can become stuck in the braces quickly.

A floss that has an end that is stiff can be used to effectively cleanse the mouth and eliminate plaque that accumulates between teeth. This floss is specially designed that has a stiffer end, it is placed between teeth. Normal floss can be difficult to use due to the wires. This floss can be used to floss.

* A waterpik device which directs high pressure water towards the teeth to remove any adhering food particles and plaque. The pressure is directed to the teeth , and it acts like floss, or a toothpick, without physically manipulating the teeth.

Treatments with fluoride can be beneficial to a teenager patient who is undergoing orthodontic treatment as they are more prone to tooth decay, based on the material they've got in their mouths. Fluoride allows for the penetration into the tissues, thereby making teeth stronger.

The tooth Decay in the elderly

For older patients tooth decay is usually more frequent. At this point the patient's overall health is drastically less ill and they might suffer from a range of health conditions that may cause more problems.

Teeth Decay and Prosthetics

Prosthetic teeth are usually linked to aging, since many people who wear dentures are old individuals. The need for dentures as they age is a common occurrence for those who were victimized by cavities in their early years. This means that the lifespan of their teeth decreases. Many of them have had the dental procedure of fillings for their teeth, root canals, or crowns, only to end up with the need for a tooth extraction, which requires tooth replacement.

Dental tooth fillings as well as root canals can quickly save a tooth's existence after being infected by bacteria. Unfortunately, these procedures can cause failure, and an examination of the appropriate prosthetic can be beneficial for older patients:

A. Removeable dentures: A simplest option for losing teeth can be removable teeth. This kind of tooth replacement is extremely conservative and rely on the form and quantity of remaining teeth and bone for support and retentiveness.

b. Dental bridges: The simplest prosthetic device that is fixed to replace the loss of a tooth will be the dental bridge. In order for a bridge to be made, the abutment or supporting teeth are removed or fabricated by a few millimeters, and then the bridge is positioned over the teeth.

C. Dental Implants: The current most reliable tooth replacement solution is to put in dental implants that function as a screw. It is designed to replace the tooth's root, to ensure that the crown can be inserted over it. The implants behave as an actual tooth, allowing permanent support can be offered without the use of any existing teeth.

d. Implant-Supported Dental Implants: If the patient is totally toothless and has no teeth remaining, a fully removable denture can be recommended. In order to increase the retentiveness of the dentures even when bone quality is low implants are put in and are incorporated into the design.

Foods: Foods to avoid and what to eat

The foods and drinks you consume can affect your well-being and condition that your mouth is in. Many people are foolish enough to ignore the fact that food doesn't matter however it is. The foods and drinks you consume affect the dental health of your mouth. If you're committed to keeping the bacterial invade out of your mouth, you should be aware of the best and worst foods to consume.

Foods to avoid:

1. Sweets Sweets and sugars are the primary causes in tooth loss. This includes all types of sweets and drinks that are sugary. They should be eliminated from your diet completely or eliminated as much as you can if you truly would like for your dental health and teeth healthy.

2. Dried Fruits: Although they belong to the category of food items that could be beneficial for oral health dried fruits like the apricots, raisins and prunes contain a lot of sugar and are, by nature, are extremely sticky. These fruits are loaded with fibers containing cellulose, which

hold sugars inside the tooth and promote the development teeth decay.

3. Foods that are sticky: They cause tooth decay due to the fact that they can easily adhere to teeth and then hide in the fissures and grooves and allow bacteria to flourish within these spaces. Some examples of food items in this category are cookies cakes and pies, pretzels potato chips and breads. They adhere to the surfaces of teeth and are difficult to remove, which is why they often reason for tooth decay.

4. Ice: Many people enjoy eating Ice. They grab a block of ice and then break it up into pieces by biting it. While it is enjoyable, but it's extremely dangerous since it could cause small tooth cracks. These tiny cracks, while fairly harmless, are transformed into places that are ideal to collect food. Food particles that are stuck in the teeth cause bacteria to grow and create larger problems.

Things to Eat and Drink:

1. Milk milk is a healthy source of calcium, which is beneficial for teeth and bones. Drinking milk will provide your teeth with the highest amount of calcium to help to prevent tooth decay and gum disease. It is possible to drink milk as a drink on its own, but you also can enjoy milk with fruits such as in smoothies and shakes or even in processed form in cheese or various dairy-based products.

2. Fish It is a fantastic supply of Vitamin D. Vitamin D is vital because it helps in an effective absorption process for Calcium making sure it isn't discarded as waste, instead, it's effectively digested through the digestive system. Fish that are fatty, such as mackerel and salmon are rich in Vitamin D. Consuming enough of these will strengthen your teeth and guard them from tooth decay.

3. Water: The best drink you can drink and is completely dental-friendly is water. Water regulates the amount and quality of saliva which assists in washing away food particles and keeps the mouth free of plaque. Hydration is crucial since saliva is

your most effective defense to tooth decay. If you are of the opinion that water is boring for your tastes, you can enhance the flavor by adding mint and lemon to your drink.

4. Nuts. Nuts aren't only natural cleanser, they also provide a healthy snack to be enjoyed because they're rich in Vitamin D and calcium , both of which is beneficial for the gums and teeth. Almonds, in particular, are high in calcium. Cashews are excellent for saliva production. Nuts are high in all kinds of minerals like iron.

5. Fruits are not only that are rich in Vitamin C which aids in the health of your gums and strengthen them Also, fruits are good due to its high amount of water, that aids in saliva formation. Fruits are also natural cleanser because of their firmness and crunch.

Although the foods you should avoid aren't necessarily harmful to your health, it is recommended to consume them in moderate amounts. Indulging too much in these foods can be hazardous So, make sure you be mindful of your consumption of sweet and sticky food items. Beware of the harmful and focus on the good things for your body and smile.

Chapter 12: Symptoms And Signs Of Teeth Decay

If you spot these signs that you have tooth decay it's recommended to speak with your dentist as soon as you notice signs of tooth decay.

When a tooth is beginning the process of decaying, it might not be able to notice any symptoms initially. As the decay progresses but you'll begin to be able to notice certain symptoms and signs.

You will know that you have dental decay when notice the following symptoms of caries:

* White streaks on enamel

* gray, brown, or black spots that stain the surface of the tooth

* tiny pits or holes on the surfaces of your teeth.

* pain or sensitivity, particularly to food or drinks which are cold, hot or sweet

* a dull pain

* slight or sharp pain particularly when you bite your nails

The gums may be inflamed, which is a sign of abscessed teeth.

* bad breath

* a bad taste in the mouth

The causes and effects of tooth Decay

Tooth decay develops over time. It is caused by specific kinds of bacteria present within your mouth.

The microorganisms are attracted by sugar. If you consume sugary foods and drinks (candy cookies, sweets, soda juice, etc.) and others) Some of the sugar remains in your mouth. If you're not able to eliminate the sugar, bacteria consume it and create acids that cause harm to your teeth, including the outer enamel and the inner dentin.

Bacteria create plaque, a sticky layer that accumulates over your tooth. It is common to find plaque in particular areas - between your teeth and around bridgework fillings, close to the gum line, as well as in the pits, grooves or fractures of the back of your teeth. If you don't remove the plaque as it becomes soft, it will be more rigid, and hard to eliminate.

The acidity of plaque damages the minerals in the outer layer that covers your teeth. The wear and tear of the enamel leads to tiny holes that may become larger with time. As the cavity gets bigger and the bacteria begin to attack them, they reach the dentin, which is the second layer, which is less brittle and less able to resist. The acids then get onto the pulp or inner tooth structure where nerves and blood vessels are located.

Dental decay that is advanced causes extreme tooth sensitivity and toothache. The pulp can be inflamed, and then abscess, creating a pus-filled pocket that is an indication of an infection caused by bacteria. It can be very painful when you bite your.

If the tooth decay gets to be extreme, you could suffer from complications. The discomfort is likely to affect your daily routine. The pain could become too intense that you be unable to focus on your job.

It can be difficult to chew food or drink. This could lead to nutritional issues or weight loss issues.

As decay progresses it is possible that you will loss your teeth. It will impact the appearance of your teeth - and in the end, it will affect confidence and self-esteem.

Risk Factors in Tooth Decay

Everyone can suffer from tooth decay. However, research shows that certain factors which can increase your chances of getting tooth decay.

If you don't take care to brush your teeth.

If you don't brush your teeth after eating or drinking and drink, plaque has the chance to grow quickly and initiate the initial stages of tooth decay.

* You don't get enough fluoride.

Fluoride is a mineral that occurs naturally recognized for its capability to prevent cavities. It is also able to reverse tooth decay, which is only beginning to show signs.

Many water providers include fluoride in their water. A lot of manufacturers of mouth rinses and toothpastes also include fluoride in their products.

Be sure that the mouth products for oral care you use include fluoride to help combat cavities.

You do not pay enough attention to teeth that are at risk of tooth decay.

The place of the tooth can affect tooth decay. The front teeth are more smooth and are easier to wash. Premolars and molars which are often called"back teeth," are most susceptible to decay. They are harder to clean and reach. They are brimming with grooves and crannies which trap food particles. Plaque builds quickly between the teeth behind and can produce acids that cause tooth enamel to be destroyed.

* You enjoy certain foods and drinks.

Do you regularly drink juices and soda? Do you enjoy ice cream milk, honey, and ice-cream? Do you consider sugary breads, cookies and cakes a included in your daily diet? Do you frequently snack on dried fruit and chips? Do you have an habit of sucking gum mints or hard candy?

The drinks and foods you consume are high in sugar, which can stay on your teeth. Your saliva is unable to remove the sugar.

You often snack or drink sodas.

Drinking or eating regularly gives the mouth bacteria constant fuel to make the acids that damage your teeth.

* You're at an age that is "right" old.

Research has shown dental decay can be more prevalent in older or younger people. Teenagers and children are most at risk of dental cavities. As are adults of a certain age.

If you are the parent of a child avoid giving his bedtime drinks with milk or juice that contains sugar. Sugar will remain on your child's teeth while they sleep. This is why you should make sure that your toddler isn't allowed to wander around drinking sweet juice or milk from a sippy cup whenever you want. This can lead to teeth decay that is early.

As you get older your gums begin to receding and your teeth become less durable. The risk of developing tooth decay. You could also be taking more preventive medications that can reduce how saliva flows. The less saliva you drink increases the chance of getting cavities.

* The dental fillings on your devices are wearing out.

Dental fillings are prone to be damaged, weaken or create rough edges as time passes. This allows plaque to build up and is harder to get rid of. The fitting of your dental appliances may alter as time passes. If they don't fit properly the decay can start at the base of their teeth.

The teeth grind.

When you grind the teeth while you're asleep or when you're under a lot of tension, you are laying your teeth exposed to decay. By grinding your teeth, you strip off the enamel's protective layer.

* You have dry mouth.

Saliva removes food particles off your teeth. It assists in removing soft plaque. It has a few ingredients which neutralize the acidity of bacterial plaque and assist in the repair of tooth decay at the beginning.

Treatments for the head or neck, certain chemotherapy medications, specific medical conditions, as well as some drugs can result in diminuting saliva production. Dry mouth is a result, which increases the risk of tooth decay.

You are suffering with eating problems.

The eating disorder known as anorexia hinders saliva production. The frequent vomiting (vomiting) which is a sign of bulimia, on contrary, causes stomach acid to run away the teeth and break down the enamel. The eating disorders that cause these problems could lead to serious tooth decay.

* You are suffering due to GERD (Gastroesophageal Reflux Disorder) as well as heartburn.

The acid or reflux that is released from the stomach can flow all over your teeth, causing damage to your enamel.

Dental Treatments for Teeth Decay

What are the best ways to treat tooth decay?

The dentist will assess how serious the decay is prior to recommending the correct dental treatment. There are a variety of treatments available:

* Treatment with Fluoride

When the tooth decay only just beginning to show signs of progress, your dentist might recommend fluoride for helping to strengthen the enamel. Professionally-prepared fluoride treatments are more powerful than the fluoride that you obtain from fluoridated tapwater or the mouth washes that are available on the market or toothpastes that you purchase. It can be in the form of a foam or gel, liquid or varnish. The dentist can either apply the treatment on your teeth or place it into a tiny tray that can be placed over your teeth.

* Dental Filling

If the decay is severe The dentist can perform dental fillings or restorative work to fill the cavities. The dentist can use composite resins, porcelain or silver amalgam for fillings.

* Crown

If you have extensive tooth decay or damage, the dentist could decide to give the dental crown. It is a custom-fitted, customized jacket designed to replace the complete original crown on the tooth that has been damaged.

In order to make the crown, your dentist will take out all decayed and damaged parts from the teeth. They may also extract portions of the healthy parts of the tooth in order to ensure an ideal fitting crown. Resin or porcelain, gold or a combination of gold and porcelain are typically used to construct dental crowns.

* Root Canal

Your dentist can decide to create an appointment for a root canal if the tooth's decay has affected the pulp, the inside that is inside the tooth. The root canal can repair and can save a severely damaged or damaged teeth in lieu of removing the tooth completely.

The dentist will take out the pulp of your tooth that has become rotten. He will then place medications to the root canal to treat infection, if needed. The dentist will then replace the pulp using an infill.

* Tooth Extraction

In some cases, the tooth can be so severely decayed there is no way to save it. The dentist could decide to extract the tooth. If you've had an extracted tooth there will be gaps that make it more likely for the remaining teeth in the mouth to change. To prevent this from happening possibility, you can choose to get a dental implant, or bridge to replace the portion of your tooth that has been taken out.

Chapter 13: Practical Strategies To Prevent Tooth Decay

If you're trying to prevent dental decay, you have a variety of preventive measures you can adopt.

Dental hygiene is the first protection against tooth decay. You can reduce the danger of plaque by cleaning and flossing your teeth consistently. If you don't remove plaque immediately the plaque will develop into tartar, and then become harder to remove.

Maintain a consistent and exact approach to your routine for daily oral hygiene.

You can reduce the amount of plaque buildup in your mouth if you provide your teeth with the care they require. Make sure to brush your teeth two or 2 times each daily. Be sure to brush every each day. If you are unable to floss your teeth following a meal, be sure you thoroughly rinse your mouth using water to rid it of the majority of food particles that are in your mouth.

Using floss allows you to remove food particles that are resistant to brushing. Flossing lets you effectively cleanse between your teeth, thereby decreasing the chance of developing gum disease and cavities.

Fluoride is required to ensure your teeth are healthy. It helps reverse tooth decay that is mild. It blocks bacteria to create acids. It stops tooth enamel from decay and also replaces the loss of minerals.

Fluoride can be used in numerous ways. It is possible to drink fluoridated water. You can also use an oral rinse with fluoride.

You can also make use of fluoride toothpaste.

Acids in your teeth can cause tooth decay. Saliva neutralizes and removes the acids, thereby preventing dental caries. You can increase saliva production when you chew gum.

Choose chewing gum that is sugar-free. Make sure you choose gum that has xylitol, which is a sugar substitute that neutralizes acids in many ways. The xylitol ingredient reduces the amount bacteria present in your mouth. It stops those bacteria that are still producing acid. It also aids your teeth naturally remineralize.

You can chew sugar-free gum in between your routine of flossing and brushing when you're out and about. It's also a great method to refresh your breath.

Make use of the mouthwash prescribed by your doctor.

Utilizing a mouthwash that is available over the counter is a great way to wash your mouth and allow it to keep it clean and fresh. You can also opt for an antibacterial mouthwash, and then raise the bar in keeping the quantity of bacteria in your mouth at bay. Your dentist may even suggest a powerful antibacterial rinse for your mouth to treat gingivitis, and speed up the healing process of painful or inflamed gums , if required.

Make sure you choose the right oral hygiene products.

Pick a toothbrush with soft bristles. Select a model that is designed for deep cleaning.

Use toothpaste that has fluoride. Fluoride strengthens teeth.

Make use of antibacterial mouthwashes to lower the levels of bacteria present in your mouth.

Chew gum containing the ingredient xylitol, which helps to stop the growth of bacterial.

Cleanse your teeth thoroughly.

It is vital to brush your teeth on a regular basis if you wish to keep your teeth healthy.

Keep a routine of brushing. It is best for you to clean your teeth at the end of each meal. This might not be feasible for all people, but. If you are unable to achieve this, you should at the very least brush your teeth twice each day, after breakfast and before the time of sleeping.

Make it an integral part of your bedtime and morning routine. Integrate it into your routine until it becomes an habit. Cleaning your teeth only takes some minutes, and it is an easy habit to develop.

The size and shape of your toothbrush are a personal preference. The majority of dentists suggest an electric toothbrush that has the shape of a round.

Use an effective toothbrush that cleans your teeth. Replace it every three months to make sure that the bristles are strong and effective. If your toothbrush gets damaged prior to when you're scheduled for replacement, don't be hesitant to purchase a brand new one as soon as you can. Bristles that are frayed do not serve any purpose in cleaning your teeth.

What amount of toothpaste should you make use of? Dental professionals say toothpaste that is the dimensions of peas is enough. Select a fluoride toothpaste that is accepted as a part of the American Dental Association.

While brushing your teeth ensure you clean all surfaces of your tooth. Place your toothbrush at a 45-degree angle towards your gums as well as your teeth. Only apply only enough pressure. When you brush your teeth, excessive force and enthusiasm could cause harm to the gums. Additionally, it can cause the bristles break up quickly.

Start by rubbing the outer surface of your teeth on the front. Do small side-to-side strokes. Then, brush the inside of the surface. Use the brush vertically, and scrub the surface with upward and downward strokes.

Then, move to those chewing surfaces on your lower and upper back teeth. Don't forget to brush along your gum line too. It is essential to brush your tongue to ensure you can get rid of any bacteria and freshen your breath.

After you have cleaned your teeth, make sure you use the right mouthwash for washing. A mouthwash that is fluoridated helps to prevent tooth decay, decreases the accumulation of plaque and helps prevent gingivitis-related diseases. Make sure that the mouthwash you use does not contain alcohol since alcohol can tend to dry your mouth. Bacteria thrive faster in dry mouth.

You should floss your teeth regularly.

You must include flossing into your routine of oral care. Even if it is an habit of brushing your teeth every day, you must floss regularly to make sure you're in a position to remove any food particles, particularly the ones that go in between your teeth.

It can be difficult to remove food particles that become stuck between teeth, such as corn-on-the cob and popcorn. It can also be difficult to get rid of food particles that become trapped under the gums. Flossing can help you get to these areas where toothbrushes can't reach.

What is the proper method to use dental floss?

Take a small piece of dental floss approximately 18 inches in length. A long length will ensure that there is enough floss available to cleanse every tooth. You should wrap a significant portion of floss around your middle finger on your right hand. Then, wrap the tail of the second edge, around that middle finger on your left.

Place the floss gently in between the teeth. Secure it between your forefinger as well as your thumb. The area should be cleaned by slipping the floss between your teeth using gentle movements of back and forth. Be careful not to press the floss against your gums.

Once you are at the line of your gum, shape your floss in a circle, keeping it in place to the tooth. Run the floss lightly against the tooth's side. tooth, move it up and down and then move it across to bring it across to the other side of the tooth. Slide it up and down then bring it back to the original tooth. Repeat this procedure through all your teeth. Make sure you continue to weave the dirty areas of floss around your fingers as you move down.

If you are unable to move a piece of floss in between the teeth you could try using the dental floss flick or floss pick. The flosspick is small plastic piece of equipment that has a tiny piece of floss is connected. The way to use a floss pick is similar to how you use string floss.

It is also possible to use an alternative water pick. The device helps remove food that has become trapped between the teeth as well as plaque, by pouring out a flow of water over the region.

Prevent dry mouth.

Dry mouth, also known as Xerostomia, is a condition caused through a variety of causes, including medical conditions or the taking prescription drugs. If your mouth gets dry and persistently dry due to these causes, you are likely to suffer from tooth decay. It will be difficult to make enough saliva to clean away food particles. The oral bacteria is more likely to flourish within your mouth.

Your dentist can suggest the best products to treat dry mouth. There are prescription as well as over-the-counter mouth rinses specifically designed to treat dry mouth.

It is also possible to suck mints, cough drops or lozenges to increase the production of saliva. Make sure the items don't contain sugar.

There are products that work for the mouth in the same way that eye drops aid in treating dry eyes. They assist in moisturizing the mucous membranes of the mouth to keep your mouth moist and neutralize the acid that causes tooth decay.

If you're suffering from a serious dry mouths, the physician may prescribe medications such as Evoxac (cevimeline) as well as Salagen (pilocarpine) in order to treat the problem.

Follow the proper dietary habits to protect your teeth from decay.

Make sure you eat foods that will ensure your teeth are sturdy and healthy. These include foods that are high in calcium, vitamins and minerals, such as eggs, cheese fresh fruits and veggies.

Avoid eating too many sweets and beverages that are sugary. The sugar they contain fuels the process of tooth decay.

Stop the habit of regularly snacking. If you eat a lot it allows the oral bacteria to produce more acid , and expose your teeth to constant acid attack.

Drink regularly throughout the day. The water will clean your mouth and stimulate saliva production to counteract the acid.

Make wise choices about your snacks. Certain types of drinks or food could accelerate tooth decay. Avoid hard candy as well as sweet treats such as cookies and cakes. Take a bite of fruit instead of cakes.

If you want an indulgence in sugar at times you can indulge by incorporating the sweet treat in your dinner. It is more likely that you produce saliva when you consume the entire meal, which can help to shield your teeth from the bacterial acids.

Beware of sweet fruit juices as well as chocolate milk and coca-colas. The sugar content in these drinks can linger on your teeth, which can lead into tooth decay. Don't drink anything other than water prior to you go to bed.

Ask your dentist to provide dental sealants.

It is simple to eliminate food particles and plaque from the areas of your teeth that are even and smooth. However, the regions of your teeth where you chew food are the most susceptible for tooth decay. These teeth are characterized by grooves and pits that allow plaque to build up and for bacteria to multiply. It's also hard to utilize a floss or toothbrush to get into all grooves to remove the food debris and plaque.

Your dentist might recommend using dental sealants in order to solve the difficulty of cleaning difficult to clean teeth like molars and premolars.

A dental sealant acts as a protective coating that guards grooved regions such as the molars and premolars from decay. It is made of soft resin to prevent bacteria from getting into these vulnerable regions. It prevents bacteria from growing in these areas , leading to tooth decay. It seals the crevices, thereby protecting teeth from decay.

Ask your dentist to design you a nightguard for your teeth.

If you're inclined for grinding the teeth during your sleep or are feeling pressure or pressure, ask your dentist if could use a nightguard to safeguard your teeth.

Visit your dentist regularly.

It is a good idea to see your dentist on a regular basis even if there are no evidence or signs of decay. If tooth decay begins it is possible that you are not aware of the initial symptoms. A dentist will be able to spot the trouble spots and help prevent the decay from progressing into something more serious. The dentist will be able to tell you what steps you should follow to be able to avoid or prevent cavities.

It is important to attend appointments for the dental appointment every two years. Dental visits regularly provide a great opportunity to discuss the most effective dental health habits, get preventive care, and help you feel comfortable when it comes to regular dental care. Once you've finished your appointment, make it an effort to make the next one.

If you are experiencing sensitivity or pain, make sure you don't delay in making an appointment with your dentist.

Healthful and nutritious foods and drinks

Like many people, you're probably aware from now on that you must to reduce your consumption of sweets such as cookies and candy for the sake of preventing tooth decay.

Your choices regarding your food have a greater impact than this when it comes to stop tooth decay. Certain foods can keep your teeth healthy and strong while others can cause tooth decay.

Delicious Foods and Drinks that are helpful

What foods are the best to keep your teeth healthy?

* Calcium

If you do not obtain enough calcium from your diet, you're more likely to get tooth decay. If you eat food that is high in calcium, it makes up a part of plaque which adheres on your teeth. It neutralizes the negative consequences of acids within the plaque. It also stimulates immediately the strengthening of and rebuilding of the tooth enamel.

Dairy is a great food source for calcium. The yogurt, cheese, as well as milk, are high in calcium. They also supply Vitamin D along with phosphates that are essential to maintain your dental health. It is possible to choose low-fat yogurt as well as skim milk if you are looking for calcium-rich alternatives that are low in fat.

Studies show that the casein in cheese is a powerful protector properties that help strengthen teeth and helps prevent cavities. Research has also shown that when eating cheese, levels of calcium in your saliva rise, which helps remineralize your teeth, and also prevent tooth decay.

Many people are not a fan of the flavor of milk. Others are lactose-intolerant. If you suffer from these issues it is possible to choose soymilk and juices that contain calcium. These products can supply users with the calcium you normally get from drinking milk.

Nuts such as Brazil almonds, nuts, and pistachios are all high in calcium. As are dried beans as well as other legumes. Bok Choy, broccoli and other leafy vegetables have calcium. Fish is a good source of calcium. You may want to consider eating canned fish that has bones to add some flavor.

* Fiber

Consuming a diet high in fiber fruits and vegetables stimulates saliva flow. The saliva contains traces of calcium and phosphate and is a powerful minerals defense that protects against cavities.

Saliva is a great way to clean your teeth, eliminating food particles. Saliva can also counteract the harmful consequences of the acids and enzymes on your teeth.

You can choose to buy fresh fruits such as oranges, apples, or bananas as well as dried fruits such as raisins, figs, cranberries or dates. Peanuts, beans, peas almonds, oatmeal along with Brussels sprouts are other high-fiber choices. Crisp carrots, crisp celery and apples are all great alternatives if you're suffering from cravings.

* Whole Grains

The iron and Vitamin B complex are essential to keep your gums in good condition. Also, magnesium is essential for healthy teeth and bones. Whole grains are high in minerals like iron and B vitamins and magnesium. They also contain high levels of fiber.

Whole-grain pasta , cereals, bran, as well as brown rice are great source of all-grain.

* Chewing Gum Sugar Free

After a snack or meal, it is possible to chew gum to remove harmful acids in food and to protect enamel. Be sure to ensure that the gum isn't laced with sugar, which can cause tooth decay.

Sugarless chewing gum has xylitol. Bacteria are not able to eat the xylitol in order to develop. It is also not metabolized to produce acids. In fact, Xylitol inhibits the development of Streptococcus mutans which is the bacterium that causes tooth decay. It also prevents the build-up of plaque as well as tooth decay.

You can utilize xylitol in its gum or mint form. It is recommended to use it three to five times daily to get the best results. Make sure that the mint or gum that you purchase contains the xylitol ingredient first. This means you can be sure that the quantity of xylitol present in the product is adequate to in preventing tooth decay.

* Tea

Tea is a great source of compounds that inhibit the development in plaque-causing bacteria. It is recommended to take a cup of green or black tea to prevent tooth decay and gum disease which these bacteria cause.

To increase the potency in your cup, make use of fluoride water for brewing it. Be sure to not add sugar to sweeten your tea , lest you degrade its antibacterial properties.

* Water fluoridated

Drinking water that is fluoridated helps improve the health of your teeth. If you prepare juice using powder or soup made from the dehydrated food items, make sure you're using fluoridated water. If you don't are able to access fluoride-containing water from your tap then you may want to consider the possibility of taking fluoride supplements.

* Wine

Wine fights off the bacteria that cause tooth decay. It contains antioxidants that are active Proanthocyanidins, particularly, that aid in keeping teeth strong and healthy.

Dangerous Foods and Drinks

As there are food items which help keep your teeth strong and healthy However, there are some food items that can cause tooth decay. You must avoid those "bad people."

* Sweet Treats

Beware of eating sugary snacks and sweets, specifically ones which are stuck to your teeth, such as lollipops, hard candy caramels, jelly beans and others. They prevent saliva from washing sugar from your mouth.

Cookies and cakes contain a significant amount of sugar which can cause tooth decay. If you've got an addiction to sweets and can't avoid these sweets be sure to reduce your intake. Opt to enjoy your sweets at specific times; avoid eating all day. Cleanse your teeth after you've enjoyed them, or carefully rinse your mouth in order to remove any leftover sugary particles that remain inside your mouth.

* Refined Carbohydrates

Foods with refined starch such as pasta, crackers chips, and crackers are as harmful for the teeth of your children as sugary sweets. They are all made of white flour. They're made up of simple carbohydrates, which are broken down into simple sugars, which the bacteria in your mouth eat to create the acids which result in tooth decay. Furthermore, foods with starch like potato chips or soft breads can get stuck in your mouth or get trapped between your teeth, causing damage on your dental.

* Carbonated drinks

Sodas are a great source of sugar. They also contain carbon and Phosphorus that stain and degrade enamel of teeth.

Iced tea, lemonades in bottles and energy drinks aren't only loaded with sugar. They also contain the highest levels of acidity that damages the enamel of your teeth.

If you have to drink these drinks then you might want to consider using straws to ensure that the sweet drink is not in close the teeth.

* Fruit Juices

Fruits are an integral element in your daily diet. However, juices from fruits could cause some problems. Fresh fruits are full of sugar and fiber. Fruit juices that are sold in the market are typically made with additional sugar to enhance their taste. They can also contain phosphoric and citric acids that can harm your teeth.

* Acidic Fruits

Lemons, like citrus fruits, contain high levels of acidity, which can cause harm on your tooth.

Chapter 14: Where Conventional Dentistry Excesses

Our teeth are made to be durable and endure for the rest of our life. The bones that we have in our teeth in case you weren't aware of that. Our teeth don't are failing us, it's us who suffer from our teeth. This can happen by two methods. The first is that drinking and eating foods that constantly weaken our teeth, making them more susceptible to the growth of bacteria and cavities, which can lead to and tooth decay. When we are more mindful regarding what we ate and consumed, we would not have dental issues.

What kinds of foods are harmful to our teeth? Anything that is high in sugar or highly acidic is harmful for your teeth. Foods such as pickles, hard candy, white bread apple, soda jelly, peanut butter and even salad dressings are extremely harmful to your teeth. Even if you believe they're "healthy" to eat, such as apples, they're not great for your teeth.

Apples, for instance, are extremely acidicand they can break down the enamel of your teeth. Therefore, drinking plenty of fluids when you consume an apple or washing your mouth after eating it with mouthwash will help keep the enamel from deteriorating. We're not telling you to consume acidic food but you should be conscious of what they're capable of and be aware of the appropriate precautions to take and ensure that you protect your teeth accordingly.

However, coffee is an unwise choice for drinking. Our husbands and me had to discover this lesson the hard way as well. Coffee isn't a cause of teeth decay. However, it could make those gorgeous pearly whites to become less attractive after a while. Let's face it, the majority of us don't drink our coffee in black which means that based on how you drink your coffee, there might be added sugars that must be considered. The sugars are an expense to our teeth as well. The stains that are not pretty due to coffee, as well as the added sugar that contributes to tooth decay, led me to reduce my coffee consumption quite a bit years ago.

Okay, so it's probably the best time to take in a glass of wine as well. Alcohol isn't the most beneficial thing for our teeth, either. Drinking a glass of wine every now and again will not harm your teeth. Drinkers who are light do not have any concerns. However, people who drink more be able to notice that over time, there is less saliva. The body produces saliva to aid in the health of our mouths. If there isn't enough saliva, individuals are at an increase risk of tooth dental decay as well as gum diseases.

Popcorn is a popular snack in the theater However, most dentists will not touch it since they are aware. Popcorn is harmful to your teeth due to it getting trapped between them and regardless of how old or old-fashioned we are , and no matter how many times we've been instructed, we all love to chew and bite on the kernels that haven't been popped. Unpopped kernels can cause a lot of trouble and we're trying to chip or break teeth when we chew on the kernels. If you decide to snack on popcorn, be sure to clean your teeth following the meal and don't forget to floss!

Like apples, citrus fruits, such as the ones mentioned above contain lots of acidity that can be harmful to your teeth. As with apples, they are extremely beneficial in different ways, making it challenging to eliminate out eating habits completely. Make sure to consume these fruits with plenty of water. Many people these days prefer to add flavor to their water using various citrus fruits, too. This can be achieved by using various varieties of essential oils rather than the fruits by themselves. It is much better than using the fruit for the acid purpose, yet will still provide you with the taste of citrus fruits that you like.

Do you remember back in the first chapter, I mentioned that our teeth fail us by two different ways? Here is another method by which our teeth fail us. We

133

damage our teeth by relying on conventional dental care to look after the condition of our teeth when in reality the responsibility lies with us to take care for their health. Traditional dentistry is a business and even though I'm not trying to claim that dentists are scam artists but they're in business to make money. When we encounter an issue in our teeth, such as discoloration or pain and pain, we rush to the dentist since it is what society was taught by us. We can spend hundreds or thousands of dollars having your dental issues "fixed" in the dentist's office , believing that filling cavities or placing crowns into our teeth can solve problems.

The same is true for two-yearly teeth cleanings. We pay for our teeth to be professionally cleaned but is it really necessary to be able to have professional cleaning done? Are we paying for other parts of our body professionally cleaned two times a year? Dental insurance companies typically cover these bi-annual cleanings as they're considered preventative. If you are able to get dental hygiene services at minimum once every year, you're less likely to require more costly work. It's the idea, at least you're thinking, right?

Why are there so many people who need dentures or are suffering from cavities each time they visit the dentist? Are there too many people who have bad dental hygiene? I am a believer with pretty good dental hygiene. I brush twice daily as well as floss three times per week. I was diligent with my routine cleanings even while we were insured. I'm not even a bit of an indulgence in sweets however, I did get cavities about every two or three times.

Dentists have an answer for this, too. Genetics is the reason as they have always said to me. My parents would have had bad teeth, and I had the same problem, too. It was almost inevitable that I was going to be a bad person and I could prefer to accept the fact that I would soon be filled with dental cavities, crowns and, eventually, dentures.

Did I already see evidence of this genetic trait being passed down to my daughter as early as the age of 3? In my opinion, this didn't make sense. There must be an option to cut the chain or to decide that it shouldn't need to be this way. I felt that the dental industry was telling me things that were logical but it also convinced me of certain things which left me with no choice but to give them more money.

I kept going to the dentist every now and then, fearing they would tell me that go, I might be left with a mouth full of stained, pirate-looking teeth. I believe that dentists hold some kind of control over us, and they threaten us to pay for their services, or being viewed as a failure in the society. Can you imagine telling your friends and family that you don't visit the dentist? What do your colleagues, friends or your family members consider?

I'm sure that most people at first would consider it to be dirty, disgusting or even unsanitary that you wouldn't visit the dentist. In the past I would have sided with those who said it was. But now, I belong in a different camp. I believe there's an alternative method to look after our teeth that does not require a visit regularly to the dentist to get a standard cleaning. I don't need to worry about dental decay or cavities as is the norm in an American family, and even more important, I don't have to fret about whether my husband's employer provides dental services, what it will cost and whether we're covered because I know that my family is protected with natural, affordable better, safer, and more natural dental treatment.

DISCOVERY AND A COMMITMENT

I found my current approach to dental care quite by accident. I've said before that I conducted many hours of online research and discovered nothing I was happy with. However, while looking into the causes and the relationships between the food we consume and our own dental needs, I started to research the foods that we shouldn't consume.

This got me thinking whether, if there are certain foods that harm our teeth, then there ought to be food items that are healthy for our teeth isn't it? That set me off on the right track and set me on the path I am on today. Through combining these two simple concepts, I've made an eating plan with two components for our family, which is comprised of the foods we try to eat frequently to maintain our dental health, as well as foods we try to stay clear of to ensure that our teeth are strong and healthy. If I say to avoid this, I'm referring to. However, we haven't eliminated them out completely from our lives. For instance, one of the food items that we are trying to stay clear of is white bread since it's loaded with sugars from the process. However, if my children visit a family member's home and they are served French toast or peanut jelly and butter sandwich on white bread, I'd prefer to not to become "that child" who would say something like, "I don't eat white bread I only eat multigrain as well as wheat."

I'm sure it's not likely to harm their teeth to consume white bread every once time.

We don't keep a ton of sweet snacks and desserts in the house however it doesn't mean that the entire family doesn't have an excuse to go out to ice cream once in a while. Just make sure that we clean our teeth when we return back home.

There are other things I've learned are healthy to our dental health. This will be something we'll discuss about in detail in the next chapter. I wanted to point out that this subject is not well-known. I've never been exposed to foods that were healthy for your teeth before. I believe it's important to be aware that these food items are available and if you wish to know more about them, there is plenty of information online about them.

I was very thrilled to integrate my findings into our routines. It was a bit of a change initially, adjusting my shopping habits and giving up some of our favourites from our family and other items, but overall it was a wonderful choice for our family.

When I began this process I was chatting with a good friend who began working using essential oils. She wanted me to experiment with them however I was not convinced on the idea that oils can help with any issue. However, she was a good friend and a very persuasive one, and so I was forced to give her the chance to show me how the oils she used could work magic.

She visited me on a Sunday day to display what she'd bought. She told me stories of the people who had issues and how the oils been able to help them recover However, I was still not convinced enough to purchase any product. At times, I joked with her, asking her if she had any results on teeth.

She consulted her small guidebook, and sure enough the oils worked. She had a variety of recipes to treat different issues that involved teeth. I was shocked by what she could do such as dental whitening gum repair abscesses, oil pulling and thrush, among others.

I was intrigued to know more of the things she said about it and test a few of them as issues occurred in our household. I'm still not able to try each one as we've not had the issues that the oils and other herbs could solve (thank for the goodness!) But the ones I've tried have been amazing. They're fast-working and aren't expensive. They can be purchased at local stores for groceries or in organic food shops. I couldn't be more pleased having found this product to enhance our family's current method to treat our teeth.

The details of how it DOES WORK

What are the best foods to consume and which ones are best avoided? It all boils down to a few fundamental guidelines. I try to stay clear of refined sugars as well as all processed grains. I make an effort to buy whole foods that are not processed. We avoid quick food outlets for the greater part right now, too. We consume all whole grains organic dairy products and canned fish (like mackerel and salmon) and spinach, carrots and turnips as well as lettuce. The following list of nutrients and vitamins to take into consideration when searching for food items:

* Bioflaviniods (Vitamin P)

* Vitamin B-Complex

* Vitamin B12

* Vitamin C

* Vitamin CoQ10

Vitamin D

* Vitamin E

* Vitamin K

* Magnesium

* Silica

* Phosphorus

* Calcium

All of these minerals and vitamins can be used together to help restore and strengthen bones which is the reason our teeth exist. They also make the bones stronger. This can help to defend them against harmful drinks and foods we consume.

Fish of all kinds are excellent for supplying these nutrients. We may not have had a large amount of fish at home prior to our decision to alter our lifestyle and eat, but once I was aware of the way to live I was forced to learn how to cook different types of fish. My husband and children have all come to appreciate fish and it's one of the best things we've added to our diets to aid us on our way to.

Calcium is a crucial element to have strong and healthy teeth and many people believe that drinking milk is the sole method to obtain calcium. While milk is an excellent sources of calcium it's far from being the only source of calcium that is there. There are plenty of excellent sources of calcium around us. Some offer other health benefits in addition! Here's a list calcium-rich drinks and foods to take into consideration:

* Cheese (in two ounces, 404 mg calcium)

* Sardines (1 can provide 351 mg calcium)

*Yogurt (1 cup with 296 mg. calcium)

* Salmon (1 can provide 277 mg. calcium)

* Whole milk (1 cup with 276 mg. calcium)

* Prepared Collard Greens (1 cup 266 mg of calcium)

* Kale cooked (1 cup, 171 mg of calcium)

* Prepared Broccoli (2 cups, 120 mg. of calcium)

Being aware that we could get calcium from various sources allowed us to feel comfortable eating a variety of different foods.

Fruit is a tricky topic to talk about as, while it's rich in minerals and vitamins, it's also a source of sugars and a lot of fruits are acidic, and as we've discussed before can be harmful for your teeth. Drinking plenty of water, or eating fruits along with a dairy that is not sugared product can fight the acidity and sugar.

For instance, eating berries and peaches along with yogurt or cream could aid. Beware of eating any dried fruit and fruit that are sweet. If you're already suffering from tooth decay or are trying to prevent tooth decay, it is recommended to avoid eating fruits in as much as you can.

Let's discuss soft drinks. Soft drinks are among the most harmful drinks that have ever been invented in the world of dental care. Soft drinks are loaded with an astonishing volume of sugar which is harmful to our teeth. Soft drinks also deprive the body of vital calcium and magnesium. We've previously discussed the need for these two minerals in order to construct solid and strong teeth. If you've had a calcium-rich meal, but later decide to sip an alcohol-based drink it's a sign that you've been counterproductive. Soft drinks can be an unintended double-whammy in terms of the health of your teeth. They not only provide sugars that are harmful and toxins, but they also take away vital minerals that help strengthen your teeth.

Many people believe that drinking sugar-free or diet soft drinks will benefit them but I'm the one who has bad news on that one too. These drinks are made with artificial sweeteners , which can be as harmful to your health as. These artificial sweeteners also harm your teeth, and the soft drinks still remove calcium and magnesium. Therefore, these drinks are not superior to the conventional varieties.

Protein is a crucial component of any diet. It is crucial to realize that what we put into our bodies impacts the overall condition of our health and that includes our oral and dental health. In the past few years, we've been more aware of the things that happen on farms and in factories that process meat to our meat and poultry. To ensure that the protein you consume to remain safe and to ensure that you don't be exposed to harmful by-products be sure that your protein comes from grass-fed animals that are fresh instead of factory-farmed eggs and meats that are sourced from profit-driven businesses. Research and find out everything possible about animal to make sure that the protein you purchase comes from animals that aren't in a state of neglect or abuse prior to it making it into your supermarket.

Avoid the usual lunch meats as well as the standard bacon hot dogs, sausages, hot dogs. Instead , opt for organic options which you can be sure are superior and have no dangerous food additives.

Do not ever consume protein powders. I am sure there will occur a moment when you believe that you could have a low protein level and you think this is the best way to ensure you're getting sufficient protein, but believe me when I say that this isn't the best solution. If there's a good source of protein available so why should you choose something that can be harmful and cause tooth decay that is full of sugars and sweeteners? Instead, opt for eggs, fish, or beef to include protein in your diet instead of incorporating powders of protein into your routine.

Many people had mercury fillings in the past. The mercury fillings aren't used any more, but if were one of them, and you still have them , or don't have your fillings changed, you might need mercury detox. It takes about two weeks to cleanse your body of the mercury that is in your system. This is logical, because the reason people had to stop mercury fillings was that mercury is toxic to our body, so why would you want to cleanse your body of mercury that is in it 24 hours a day?

The detoxification process isn't very difficult, in fact. The method involves incorporating fresh cilantro to your diet every day for at least 2 weeks. Simple enough, isn't it? That's it. If you are able to manage by adding garlic or fish oil, it could be beneficial, too.

Vitamin C is a crucial element for good health and healthy teeth. Many people think of oranges or other citrus fruit when thinking of Vitamin C. True, it is true that oranges contain an adequate amount of vitamin C however, as we've mentioned previously citrus fruits aren't the best choice for your teeth due to the acidic properties of these fruits. If you're not allowed to eat citrus fruits, but you're in need of vitamin C to keep your teeth healthy How else do you obtain it? Here is a great guide to other resources of vitamin C.

* CamuCamu

* Rose Hips

* Acerola Cherry

* Red Pepper

* Parsley

* Guava

* Broccoli

* Strawberry

* Kale

* Raw Cabbage

The food and guidelines are fairly easy to follow. The guidelines aren't designed to be difficult rather, it's created to be flexible with various choices. I was able to identify the foods to stay clear of however, I also discovered the minerals and vitamins that I need to focus on including into our diets. I was introduced to these minerals and vitamins, and that's the point at which my real research began.

I started looking into food items and meals I could prepare and serve my family. I knew it would be a radical shift for us. I was aware that my kids had to learn about new foods, and eventually they would be able to stop wanting to eat their favorite foods. It took time, and the change wasn't instantaneous However, the next chapter will reveal how I integrated all of this into my daily routine.

How I made it work ME

It wasn't as easy as one three, two and a visit to the supermarket after which the new design was put into place in our home. It was a long process, spanning weeks and months later, we're still trying to adjust to the new way of life however, it's successful and we are thrilled with the result.

I'm constantly searching for new ways of cooking my food. I started by looking up an inventory of the vitamins, and then learning about the foods that contain those vitamins. It was difficult as some food items were high in vitamins, but they were not good for our teeth.

We talked briefly about citrus fruits and vitamin C and I did many inter-referencing when I first began. However, the more I played on it, the more comfortable I became. The things started to click for me. The things to avoid such as acidic food items or sugary foods, were embedded into my brain, and when I saw recipes with these ingredients I put them away or was able come up with alternatives to influence to their advantage.

I'll admit I was somewhat obsessed with spending time, with everything. It was like an enjoyable hobby to try to discover new recipes, and anything else that I needed to prepare for the family. We tried a few and loved other recipes we tested and were able to discard. It was like playing a fun game.

More importantly we noticed the improvement in our dental and oral health after a few weeks of following the new food regimen. My daughter was no longer complaining about pain in her mouth and no longer required any pain medication any more. I noticed that my mouth was gradually getting better also. After about one months, my mouth was gone.

The things weren't perfect for our family, but we don't have everything done in a strict manner. As we have embraced this new lifestyle in our family, we've removed a lot of things from our house, however we're still lax on certain things.

We do go out for take a bite to eat once or twice a month. If you do go out, let our children to select what they'd like to eat from the menu. Sometimes, they'll order soda, but sometimes they opt to have water. While I can appreciate the implications of drinking having a soft drink but I don't think that drinking it at least every 6 weeks or each month is going to cause harm to their health. Different people may be feeling differently, and to be their own however, that's how we have decided to manage the family business.

This is also true to other items as well like popcorn and candy. We don't store these in our home but when we go to the cinema or for other occasions, we're able to indulge and enjoy them. We don't feel that allowing ourselves or our children to indulge every frequently will damage your dental hygiene.

This is clearly an individual decision we , as a family, have taken and you are free the best choices in the same manner. We feel that when we do not have these types of things around the house the kids, as well as really my husband and I also, view them as a reward or treats.

Although I want it My husband and I have decided to stop drinking coffee as part of our lifestyle change. It was something we were aware of the need to do and it nearly broken my heart to make it. I was awed by getting up before the kids awoke and sipping my coffee. It was "my daytime." I created my perfect coffee by adding a small creamer, and a small amount of sugar. My coffee was perfect cup over many years and to give the cup away was the equivalent of giving up a small piece of me.

It was at first that I felt like a zombie , without my cup of morning coffee There are a variety of foods that are natural to give you an "pick you to get going." As an alternative to coffee you can try the apple or small handful of nuts. A glass of 16 ounces of chilled water can help people remain awake as the afternoon slump comes in.

As I mentioned, I was really struggling without coffee for a while but I was certain that if I could get to the end of my first week I'd be able kick my coffee addiction. The toughest part wasn't the dependence. I was able to get through the week, and then I stopped drinking coffee to get through the rest of my day. The toughest part was that I actually loved my cup of coffee. I loved the 30 or so minutes that I read my morning newspaper and waited for my children to rise. It was a part of my routine and was something I was eager to do every morning.

When I lost that portion in my life, I was not so happy. I needed to figure out how to restore that pleasure without coffee. I decided to go with something different than coffee. I had the tall glass of water instead. Although it wasn't quite as good however, I was able to take pleasure in my water glass and the peaceful morning, before the kids woke up. It took some time before I realized that it wasn't coffee that I loved more than the time, the paper and silence. I didn't require coffee to make this time memorable.

There were many changes like these that took place during the first few months . This caused the changes to be difficult and changing can be sometimes a bit difficult. However, overall, it was worth it.

Below are a few of the recipes we've tried to feed our family. It's evident that certain recipes were designed to avoid problems and others were to help to solve problems we encountered.

My husband and I disagreed regarding our preferred treatment for gingivitis and I'll be sharing both. He prefers the herbal treatment while I prefer the clove.

Clove Oil Remedies for Gingivitis

10 drops of clove oil

1 oz. olive oil, sesame oil, etc. (any food oil)

Mix the oils of clove and sesame in the dish of a small size. Then , using an Q-tip or a cotton ball, place it in the mixture and rub it on the area that is affected. This can be done at least three times per day until your pain has gone away.

Herbal Remedies for Gingivitis

1 C of ground turmeric

1 C myrrh powdered

1/2 cup of dried ground peppermint leaves

1/4 cup of cinnamon

A small amount of ground cloves

Make sure you have all the ingredients in your kitchen and mix them to create a powder. With the tooth brush, dip it into the powder, and then brush your teeth lightly. It is possible to brush your teeth as many as three times a each day. When you're done, rinse your mouth with saliva, however, do not use any water to wash your mouth.

Both my husband and me were treated with mercury fillings (does it reveal what age we are?) It was essential for us to go through the mercury detox. Here are some recipes we made to assist in this mercury cleansing. Remember that it was essential to include garlic, cilantro as well as fish oils in the diet for at minimum two weeks to assist with the detox.

Fresh Cilantro Salsa

10 cloves of garlic

1 C finely chopped cilantro

Four chopped, green peppers

Half C of chopped, seeded and diced tomatoes

1 C diced onion

3 T olive oil

3 1/2 3 1/2

1 1/4 1 t cumin

Salt to taste

Place the garlic in the food processor until thoroughly chopped. Add the other ingredients to the blender. Blend until smooth or until you get the desired texture. Serve with chips or as a snack with barbecued chicken, meats hamburgers, etc. Refrigerate until you are ready to serve, if not immediately.

Cilantro Pesto

1 C of fresh cilantro leaves

1/2 C almonds

3 cloves of garlic large

1/4 C grated Parmesan cheese

1/4 C olive oil

1/2 1 t salt

Chop the garlic, cilantro and almonds and put them in a food processor or blender. Blend until smooth. Add grated parmesan as well as salt and oil. Blend again until you reach desired consistency. It should end up being a smooth paste. Mix it with pasta that is hot. Serve hot.

Natural Whitening of Teeth

Strawberries

Toothbrush

Make use of strawberries and smash them into the form of a paste. Make use of your toothbrush and the strawberry paste as your toothpaste. Cleanse your teeth using the strawberries. Keep the strawberries on your teeth for as long as you can. Don't rinse your mouth.

Anti-gingivitis Sage & Myrrh Powder

1/2 C of ground sea salt

1/4 C dried horsetail

1/4 C of dried leaves of sage

1 T spearmint or peppermint leaves

10 drips of myrrh oil

Mix all the ingredients in a large bowl and mix thoroughly. Pick up your toothbrush and wet it by soaking it in water. Dip it in the mix and then scrub your teeth lightly with the mix. You could spit your saliva however, do not rinse.

Gum Tightening Cinnamon Powder

1 T bentonite clay

2T sea salt

1 T chaparral that has been dried

2 T ground cinnamon

Mix all ingredients together in a small bowl , and mix thoroughly. Use your toothbrush to wet it by soaking it in water. Dip it in the mix and then scrub your teeth lightly using the mixture. You could spit your saliva however, don't rinse.

If you believe you're fighting tooth decay, there are some foods you can include in your diet to help to repair your tooth enamel. These are foods that are high in silica which will aid in the repair and rebuilding process.

* Alfalfa

* Buckwheat

* Chickweed

* Dandelions

* Kelp

* Lamb's quarters

* Oat straw

* Oats

* Lentils

* Leaf of raspberry

* Spelt

* Sunflower seeds

*Tomatoes (Remember tomatoes are very acidic, and can harm your teeth as well! Make sure you drink plenty of water while eating them to prevent the acid from sticking to the teeth.)

When we were deciding on the essential oils and other items to help our families, most of the time we utilized the oils for my husband and myself. Essential oils aren't always safe for children, and it's recommended to keep them away from children's access into them. The solutions worked for us, including those that are preventative, and we're able to recommend these to you with no hesitation.

OFTEN ASKED QUESTIONS

Shouldn't I simply consume a multi-vitamin for the nutrients?

It's a sensible concept, but it's not the case. The majority of research indicates that the body is healthier when it gets the vitamins from natural sources instead of artificial ones. Although a multi-vitamin supplement is better than nothing, it's still not likely to provide you with the most effective results. When you find food items that provide the minerals and vitamins mentioned above, you'll provide your body and , in essence, you teeth, with ingredients they require to remain healthy and strong over a longer time.

Essential oils: What do they mean?

Essential oils are volatile oils that a plant produces.

Are essential oils safe for use by children?

Unfortunately, no. Some oils are fine, and others may be reduced to a lesser degree, and some never. It is crucial to do your own research prior to giving essential oils to your children to ensure that the oils are secure. I was unable to locate oils that I could trust with my children, specifically ones that are used for oral use, as many oils are safe only applied topically (on the surface of the body) to children. However, after changing our diet and began feeding my kids nutritious foods that aid in dental health I noticed that our oral hygiene (children inclusive) increased dramatically. All that said I'd recommend that you seek guidance from a pediatric dentist before giving essential oils younger children.

Where can I get essential oils?

Essential oils are sold nearly everywhere. They are available in the big box stores nowadays, however for the best quality products you should look for one that is 100 100% essential oil, and organic. A lot of essential oils today are used for scent or may be sold in this way which means they're packed with artificial chemicals. Beware of this and make sure to read the labels so you can be sure that you're buying a product 100 percent pure.

Do essential oils pose a risk for everyone to make use of?

Unfortunately, no. Certain essential oils are dangerous to swallow, and should be handled with attention. Essential oils should be handled with extreme caution and care particularly around children. Anyone who is currently seeking medical attention to treat any other reason is advised to consult with their doctor to determine whether the essential oils they are using are suitable to use whether orally or topically. If you're taking any prescription drugs it is recommended to talk to your doctor to make sure your essential oils do not interact with your medication negatively. Always stay on the edge of prudent.

Do essential oils pose a risk to use if I'm nursing or pregnant?

There are some that are absolutely not. It is crucial to do your research prior to doing anything drastic during pregnancy. Similar to getting an xray at the dental office can cause harm to your child as can the application of essential oils on a cavity that is healing. I would advise caution and suggest talking with your health care provider prior to taking any action or making changes within your routine. It is the same for changing your diet. While I am a firm believer in our eating habits currently, and I believe they're extremely healthy however, it isn't my job to be a physician and I only want the best for women who are pregnant and nursing mothers. Always talk with your doctor prior to making any changes like this.

What drinks can I have?

Water is the best option to protect your smile. Although I'm sure that's not what you'd like hear, but a lot of other drinks are not good to your dental health. Anything that contains sugars, or artificial sweeteners, can be harmful to your teeth. Wine, alcohol, coffee, tea, etc. do not make it into the list either. Of course, it's acceptable to indulge once the time, but be aware that they're not good for your teeth and it's best drinking them with plenty of water or at a minimum, clean your teeth as quickly as you are able after you've consumed these drinks.

TIPS and INSIGHTS

Start slow

Sometimes, the changes are dramatic and may feel incredibly extreme. Start slow and you'll feel more relaxed about the new experience and are less likely to fall back. It's not necessary to make an overnight change. Instead of throwing out the food you have and spending money on all new things, try purchasing something new and throwing out the things you're doing now to stay clear of. Try it for the duration of a week. In the beginning of the following week you can do a little purge once more. Every month, clean out a bit more and purchase some more items. When the month is up and you'll realize that you've gotten rid of everything, and your refrigerator and pantry are filled with everything you could think of.

Return to the Horse

It is inevitable that you'll make mistakes at some point or other. It's okay. Everyone has a moment of weakness and when that happens you can pick yourself up and give yourself a few words encouragement then remind yourself you'll be better the next day. Your teeth won't decay and fall out of your mouth due to the fact that you chose to indulge in one bite from chocolate cake. Brush your teeth as fast as you can and remember to floss! Make a promise to yourself that tomorrow will be the day to start again.

Recognize Your Strengths and Blow Your Strengths

Are you a sucker for chocolate cakes and citrus fruit? What is the thing that consumes you each day? If it's chocolate cake, then first be sure that there isn't any chocolate cake that is close enough to make you want to eat it. This is the same for any other weakness you may be suffering from. The weaknesses you have will be revealed fast when you begin changing your eating habits. You'll begin to crave certain foods and then you'll be able to pinpoint what your weaknesses are in case you didn't already know. Take your weaknesses out of your home. This is your first move. It's easier to get out of sight and getting out of mind. If that isn't enough to take care of the issue, seek out something else to keep you busy. Take a break from reading, watching an e-book, concentrate on your work, play a sport or. Find a way to distract you from food. If this isn't working Find a healthier snack you can consume as an alternative.

Do not cook things that are too difficult to cook.

We're not trying to dissuade people from trying out new foods however, in the beginning especially, do not try to cook food that is out of your comfort zone. I did that when I tried to master cooking fish. I had only cooked fish a few times and naturally, I considered I was a pro. I chose a recipe that was clearly labeled as advanced however, instead of ignoring the recipe's label, I tried regardless. The fish came out too cooked and the vegetables were not cooked properly. I was stunned and felt like I was a bit disappointed. Troy tried to eat the entire thing down for me however I was unable to take less than 3 bites prior to throwing it out. I'm sure Troy was happy that I threw it away. Beware of my advice, explore new recipes however cook at a level that you are comfortable with at least for some time.

Give up smoking and coffee

Two things that can't be more detrimental to your dental health than smoking cigarettes and drinking coffee. I don't know how to express how much I adored coffee, but after recognizing the dangers it could cause to the teeth of my family, I quit the habit. If you're an avid smoker or coffee drinker, follow my advice. It gets more difficult to stop, and will only harm your smile the more you hold off. You may think that you'll be able to brush your teeth, and then regularly whiten them to stop the staining, but I'm here to tell you to stop now. Your teeth will be grateful in the future.

Chapter 15: What Is The Reason For The Tooth Decay

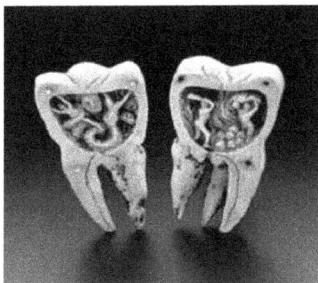

"The The Myth about the Tooth Worm...as depicted in ivory sculptures to left, was first recorded by the Sumerians in the year 5000 BC"

What is the root cause of tooth decay and dental cavities?

Diet

What I was most interested about in this query is the fact that the person asking it is only concerned with teeth, and not to nerves or gums. A lot of us are misinformed regarding bones being flexible and irreparably damaged once we are adults. If they're brittle and fixed, then we could be wondering if there's anything that we can do to treat them. Let's first look at the physical requirements of bones to stay healthy before we examine the true nature of tooth decay.

Dental geniuses have enlightened us by revealing the root causes of tooth decay. The good doctors discovered that the people from the past around the globe who consumed a lot of vegetables and fruits had no dental cavities or decay. The dentists found that the cases of tooth decay didn't appear until the diet was changed towards more agricultural foods such as sugars, flour and meats.

There are many people who suffer from an illness whose official title has been "dental caries." The disease affects about 90 percent of the people. It becomes more severe as you age. Around 28% of children between 2 and 5 years olds have dental cavities and by the time they are between the ages of 20 and 39, the percentage rises to 92 percent. The disease isn't cured with chemicals, detergents or other chemicals or by a variety of other products, and certainly not curable by dentists who drill holes into teeth.

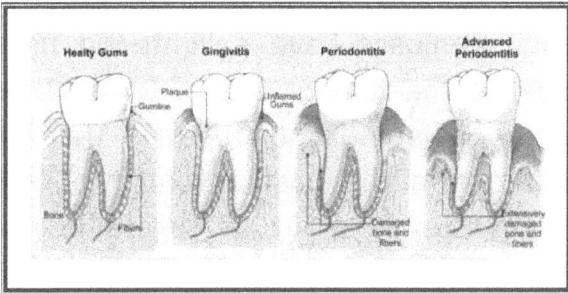

Dehydration

The human body is made up of 75 percent water. With blood being 92 percent water, bones 22, percent water and muscles 75% water. It's not surprising that our immune system is influenced by our intake of water. We are often told that drinking drinks like juices from fruit tea, soda, or tea can keep us properly hydrated and also provide water. But the truth is that these drinks actually remove water from your body since they are high in salts and sugars. Dehydration can be detrimental to teeth. It not only removes minerals from your body but removes water as well and creates toxins, which can contribute to tooth decay and formation of cavities.

Chemicals

There are a variety of pharmaceuticals found in municipal water sources. It is important to note that the U.S. Government does not need to conduct any tests for the presence of drugs in the water sources. We have only presented an analysis of two most prevalent toxins inside U.S. water supplies below. We did not consider the risks of pesticides, heavy metals as well as drugs and industrial contaminants that are common components of municipal water sources. Chlorine is the biggest stifler and killer of the present. While it slowed the spread of one disease, it also created another. Fluoride is known as a neurotoxin, which was extensively used during World War II by the Nazis to help pacify prisoners of war.

Caveman Style Modern Dentistry

Orthodontists, dentists, dental surgeons, and all of them are unable to offer a permanent natural solution to your dental problems. They can prescribe medicines and help alleviate symptoms, but they are unable to solve any issue. In fact, they can only exacerbate the dental issue while also expanding your pockets. Most people go to the dentist due to the belief that this is the place to should go if you're suffering from a dental issues. This is the current norm. People don't bother to look inside any longer. One of the examples of this bizarre normal is the mentality of how people handle the problem of wisdom teeth.

Wisdom teeth are considered to be superfluous and that's why they must be removed in the early years before they cause trouble. They are believed to be susceptible to cause an anterior tooth crowding, as well as gum infections. They can be hard to maintain clean because they're in the back of your mouth. Hence, it is important to get them removed immediately, before any problems develop. This is not the kind of an approach to thinking holistically. It's like dental professionals placing fillings into the grooves of teeth that are not carious simply because they are more likely to create cavities. This may sound absurd, but the procedure is done daily. The rational mind will tell you that all your teeth are vital with wisdom, and that includes. According to Chinese medical theory every tooth runs through meridians throughout your body, which affect the organs and other the body's components. The wisdom teeth, in particular, are linked with the heart as well as intestinal meridians. So is it any wonder that chronic illnesses in both organs is increasing? I've had the experience of having my wisdom teeth extracted in the past four years due to discomfort, however after repairing my teeth I'm grateful to have them in good health and intact. Your body will be grateful for it. I have all of my wisdom teeth even when it was strongly suggested that I extract them. I was of the opinion that life provides us with many metaphors to provide clues to the reason that we might be confronted with any obstacle or problem and if you can conduct a into the root of the motivation behind the problem it will bring us more likely to allow the issue to go away.

Chapter 16: The Way To Repair Your

Teeth

How often have we wondered what is the reason God lets suffering, pain and illness to be present in the world? Many people think that the pain they're suffering is caused by accidental events, or is caused by random bad luck "why me God what is the reason? ???? Spiritualists consider it a punishment by an a higher power due to a spiritual debt.

Many people have lost sight of the basic reality behind the significance of suffering. The basic truth that all suffering and pain is caused by self-inflicted mental trauma. The meaning behind suffering stems from the physical, emotional, and mental expression of an internal imbalance.

It is important to understand that suffering and pain have meaning in the same way as dreams are meaningful. As symbols that we see in dreams suffering and pain are messages sent by the subconscious mind, which can be understood and interpreted by paying close attention. But, the suffering and pain aren't the cause of the issue they are just a sign of the issue. The root of the problem lies within us and is caused by an unbalance in our attitudes, thinking and emotions.

In defining disease as just related to the body The medical model has diverted the minds of many people from the real cause of the illness and caused fear that only medications or other treatments can cure it. It's a phobia that shouldn't have been there in the first place. If medical treatment seems to work but it's just an interim fix, unless the actual spiritual, non-physical reason has been dealt with.

Knowing the Signs and Signals that indicate tooth problems

Toothache and/or Tooth Decay

Sign/Signal: Overeating, indigestion, digestive problems.

Meaning The reason you find it difficult to stay on track and not paying attention to your long-term requirements

Physical manifestation Dental loss and confidence in yourself. The feeling of not knowing the truth can be a sign of the choices you're not making.

Solution: It's an issue of the solar and root chakra problem. You're not connected to the world. A bad mouth is a sign that you are that you are letting your power go. Find your purpose in life and be the person who has the confidence to follow through it. It is impossible to replace you and you are worthy of being there. Spend more time in the outdoors and with those who care about you regardless of what.

Grinding Your Teeth

Sign/Signal: Frustration anger, ineffective communication skills, having not to be heard or speaking up.

Meaning: Tight teeth or headaches, a stiff neck, a limited bite, and a lack of appetite, the tension of your jaw. Teeth grinders have difficulty chewing. This could be an analogy for the life that has been squandered!

Solution Answer: This concerns the throat. problem. It's time for you to make your ideas visible. Write a diary, learn public speaking. Take note of your own voice and let your inner voice be strong in silence. Let your inner critic stop! Sing.

Bad Breath

Signal or Sign The body doesn't pay any focus on your body until it's angry with you. You're too involved in other people's issues to take care of your own. You're giving away too much, but not getting.

Meaning: People aren't likely to touch you. You feel uncomfortable and bad breath is typically an indication for tooth decay.

Solution The answer is that it's an issue with your heart chakra. Take a deep breath. You are as worthy of love as everyone else. Be aware of your heartbeat and only assist only when you are willing to. Doing otherwise is to create a system that allows others to exploit you. You must step out of your comfortable zone. You are dehydrated. Cleanse, detoxify your mind body and soul.

Natures Best Mouthwash The best mouthwash is water (distilled/spring) Charcoal, Coconut Oil, Sea Salt and organic lemons.

The Art and Science of Oil Pulling

Oil pulling is an excellent oral detoxification process that can be performed by simply shaking the coconut oil in a tablespoon or distillated water.

Oil pulling is a simple process. It is basically a matter of wash your mouth, just like you would the use of a mouthwash. It's as easy as it sounds when done properly, it can have a powerful cleansing and healing effect not just on the sinuses and mouth, but also on the whole body.

Oil pulling is traced back to the practice of oil gargling that was used in the ancient Ayurvedic medicine. Oil pulling is the act of swishing and not gargling. Oil is "worked" inside the mouth through pulling, pushing, and then dripping it down the teeth for a time between 15 and 20 minutes. The process is performed one to three times daily with a full stomach.

The oil is not taken in because it is filled with toxins, bacteria and mucous. It acts as cleanser. When you place it into your mouth and then move it into the gums and teeth the oil "pulls" out dirt and bacteria. It functions similar to the oil that you use into your car engine. The oil sifts the dirt, grime and other particles. When you empty the oil it sifts out grime and dirt and leaves the engine clean. Also, when we remove toxic substances from our bodies, our health improves and our engines run more smoothly and can last more.

Conclusion

I'm hoping that you're also able to grasp the anatomy of your teeth. By understanding this, you will be able to better comprehend how to take dental care. My primary goal to do this is to begin eating the right food choices and avoid eating food items that harm your teeth. If you do this, you'll be able to promote long-term dental health and enjoy a an attractive and healthy smile throughout your life.

It is the next stage to apply the information you've learned every day, to begin making healthier choices. Small things, such as cutting down on soda consumption, could significantly impact the health of your teeth.